Non-Surgical Hair Restoration

Hair loss is one of the most common conditions encountered in both clinical and aesthetic medicine, and its impact often extends well beyond the physical appearance of patients. While surgical restoration has traditionally garnered the most attention, the field of non-surgical hair restoration has expanded significantly—driven by advances in molecular biology, the development of new therapeutic modalities, and increasing demand for lower-risk, patient-tailored treatments.

This book was written to provide a comprehensive, evidence-based overview of non-surgical approaches to hair restoration. It is intended for clinicians, trainees, and specialists seeking a deeper understanding of the available tools and how to use them effectively.

Non-Surgical Hair Restoration

A Comprehensive Guide for Doctors

Robert Dorfman MD
Founder and Medical Director, Done by Dorfman Clinic
Founder and CEO, Hair 1000 Corporation
Beverly Hills, California

CRC Press
Taylor & Francis Group
Boca Raton London New York

CRC Press is an imprint of the
Taylor & Francis Group, an **informa** business

Designed cover image: Shutterstock

First edition published 2026
by CRC Press
2385 NW Executive Center Drive, Suite 320, Boca Raton FL 33431

and by CRC Press
4 Park Square, Milton Park, Abingdon, Oxon, OX14 4RN

CRC Press is an imprint of Taylor & Francis Group, LLC

ISBN: 978-1-032-70528-6 (hbk)
ISBN: 978-1-032-72631-1 (pbk)
ISBN: 978-1-032-72639-7 (ebk)

DOI: 10.1201/9781032726397

Typeset in Garamond
by Deanta Global Publishing Services, Chennai, India

Contents

Preface

Hair loss is one of the most common conditions encountered in both clinical and aesthetic medicine, and its impact often extends well beyond the physical appearance of patients. While surgical restoration has traditionally garnered the most attention, the field of non-surgical hair restoration has expanded significantly, driven by advances in molecular biology, the development of new therapeutic modalities, and increasing demand for lower-risk, patient-tailored treatments.

This book was written to provide a comprehensive, evidence-based overview of non-surgical approaches to hair restoration. It is intended for clinicians, trainees, and specialists seeking a deeper understanding of the available tools and how to use them effectively. The basic principles underlying hair loss and the clinical assessment of varying etiologies are discussed alongside established and emerging pharmacologic therapies and newer interventions including platelet-rich plasma (PRP), microneedling, low-level laser therapy, and energy-based devices. Additional chapters examine the role of scalp health, nutritional status, and lifestyle factors in long-term hair maintenance.

The aim of this work is not simply to list treatment options, but to offer context, highlighting when and how specific interventions are most effective, and how to integrate them into patient-centered care. In a field where outcomes are closely tied to self-perception and quality of life, thoughtful selection and sequencing of therapies matter.

Whether used as a reference or a starting point, this text is meant to support evidence-based, individualized care in a rapidly evolving area of medicine to maximize patient satisfaction and meaningful results.

Acknowledgments

I gratefully acknowledge the medical student co-authors whose research, writing, and editorial contributions greatly enhanced the quality and accuracy of this textbook. Under my mentorship, these individuals assisted in developing, reviewing, and refining the content for specific chapters. Their collaboration, attention to detail, and commitment to medical education were invaluable to this project.

Contributors

Julyssa Renteria
University of South Florida Morsani College of Medicine, Class of 2027

Hamzeh Bilal
University of Colorado School of Medicine, Class of 2028

Haley Guinan
Western Atlantic University School of Medicine, Class of 2028

Sophia Kurian
Lake Eerie College of Osteopathic Medicine, Class of 2027

Robert Greer
Founder and CEO of SovDoc Corporation

Chapter 1

Anatomy and Physiology of Hair

Bilal F. Hamzeh, Julyssa A. Renteria and Robert Dorfman

Introduction

Hair is an essential component of human anatomy, playing a significant role in protecting the scalp, regulating body temperature, and contributing to one's aesthetic appearance and psychological well-being. Understanding the intricate anatomy and physiology of hair is not just academic—it's the foundation of effective hair restoration. In my practice, I've found that a deep knowledge of hair biology allows me to pinpoint the root causes of hair loss more accurately and tailor treatments more effectively. It's like having a roadmap to each patient's unique hair restoration journey. For medical professionals specializing in hair restoration (or hoping to!), an in-depth understanding of the anatomy and physiology of hair is crucial. This chapter provides a comprehensive examination of the structure of hair follicles, the intricate processes governing the hair growth cycle, and the myriad factors influencing hair health. With this foundational knowledge, practitioners can enhance their diagnostic accuracy and therapeutic strategies in addressing hair loss.

Structure of Hair Follicles

Hair follicles are complex structures embedded in the dermal layer of the skin, responsible for the production and growth of hair. Each follicle operates as an independent unit and undergoes a continuous cycle of growth and rest. The follicle itself is composed of multiple layers and components that work synergistically to produce hair (Figure 1.1).

Layers and Components of Hair Follicles

The hair follicle is a complex mini-organ embedded within the dermis of the skin. It consists of multiple distinct layers and regions, each playing a crucial role in the hair growth cycle and its structural integrity. The follicle is composed of the inner root sheath (IRS), outer root sheath

DOI: 10.1201/9781032726397-1

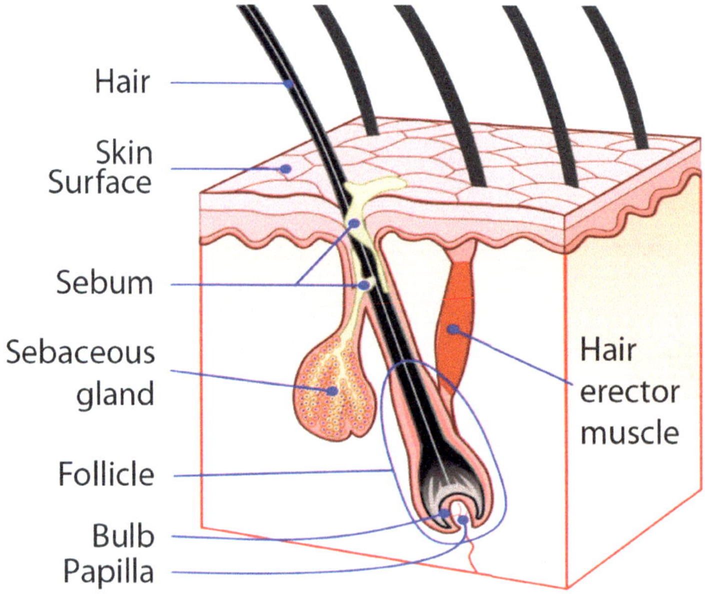

Figure 1.1 Cross-sectional diagram of hair follicle (Wikipedia, public domain).

(ORS), and surrounding connective tissue sheath (CTS) (Panteleyev 2018). These layers encase the hair shaft and provide mechanical and biochemical support. The IRS surrounds the growing hair shaft and is divided into Henle's layer, Huxley's layer, and the cuticle of the IRS, guiding the hair shaft as it emerges and disintegrating near the skin's surface. The ORS extends from the epidermis, containing keratinocytes capable of proliferating and contributing to hair regeneration while also providing structural support. The CTS, which contains fibroblasts, collagen, and elastic fibers, anchors the follicle within the dermis (Clemmensen et al. 1991).

The hair follicle can be divided into three main regions: the infundibulum, isthmus, and bulb. The infundibulum is the upper portion, extending from the skin surface to the sebaceous gland duct, facilitating the release of sebum and serving as a conduit for the emerging hair shaft. The isthmus lies between the sebaceous gland duct and the arrector pili muscle insertion site, representing the middle third of the follicle and playing a critical role in follicle integrity. At the base of the follicle, the bulb houses the dermal papilla, a cluster of mesenchymal cells essential for signaling and nourishment, and the matrix, which contains rapidly proliferating keratinocytes and melanocytes responsible for hair formation and pigmentation (Sperling 1991).

Several accessory structures are associated with the hair follicle, including the sebaceous gland, the arrector pili muscle, and a dense vascular and neural network. The sebaceous gland produces sebum, which lubricates the hair and skin. The arrector pili muscle, a small band of smooth muscle, contracts to raise the hair in response to stimuli such as cold or fear, causing "goosebumps." The dermal papilla is nourished by a capillary network, while sensory nerves surrounding the follicle provide tactile sensations (Poblet et al. 2002).

Functionally, the hair follicle operates in cycles of growth (anagen), regression (catagen), and rest (telogen), ensuring continuous hair renewal throughout life. The anatomy of the hair follicle is intricately designed to regulate these phases of the hair cycle through coordinated interactions between its components. The dermal papilla, located at the base of the follicle within the bulb, plays a central role in signaling these phases. It communicates with the matrix, a population of rapidly dividing keratinocytes and melanocytes, to sustain anagen by promoting hair shaft production and pigmentation. During catagen, the follicle undergoes apoptosis-driven regression, shrinking in size as the matrix cells cease proliferation and the dermal papilla retracts upward. In telogen, the follicle enters a quiescent state, with minimal metabolic activity, until external or internal signals, such as those mediated by hormones or cytokines, reinitiate anagen. This cyclical process is tightly regulated by growth factors, signaling molecules, and interactions between the epithelial and mesenchymal components of the follicle, ensuring balanced hair growth and shedding. As such, hair growth and loss are heavily influenced by genetic, environmental, nutritional, and other factors. Dysregulation of these cycles can lead to hair loss disorders, making the follicle a focal point for restoration therapies. Understanding its anatomy, function, and the complex interplay between follicle anatomy, activity, and other biochemical processes influenced by a plurality of factors is foundational for developing effective hair restoration treatments.

Hair Growth Cycle

When I explain the hair growth cycle to my patients (Figure 1.2), I emphasize that each phase is crucial for healthy hair growth and that various factors can disrupt this delicate balance. Hair growth is a dynamic and cyclical process characterized by three distinct phases: anagen, catagen, and telogen. Each phase is regulated by various genetic, hormonal, and environmental factors, dictating the growth, regression, and rest of hair follicles.

Anagen Phase

The anagen phase is the active growth period of the hair cycle, lasts between 2 and 7 years, and accounts for 85–90% of the hair on the scalp. During this phase, matrix cells in the hair bulb proliferate rapidly, differentiating into various cell types that form the hair shaft and root sheaths.

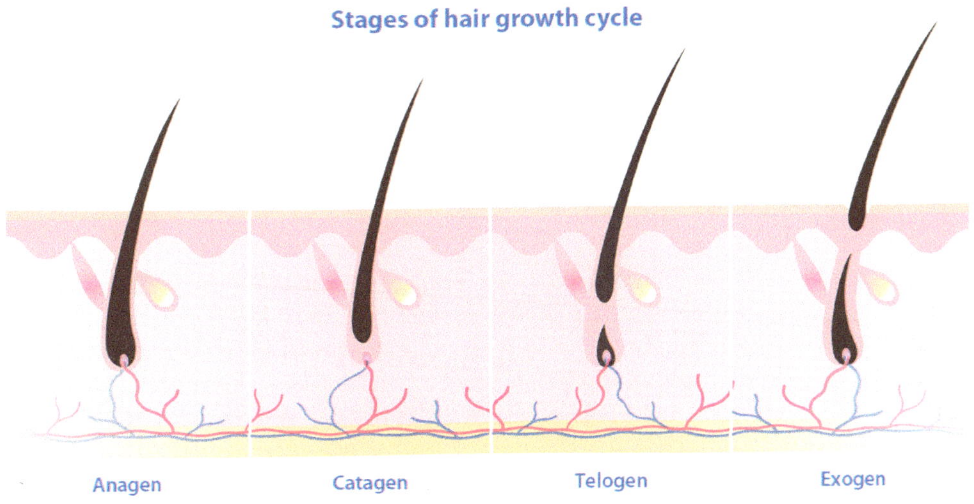

Figure 1.2 Stages of hair growth cycle (from Shutterstock, under license).

The duration of the anagen phase determines the maximum length of the hair. Factors such as genetics, health status, and hormonal balance influence the length of this phase. Hair follicles in the anagen phase are deeply embedded in the dermis, and the dermal papilla provides continuous nourishment and growth signals. In patients with hair loss conditions, such as androgenetic alopecia, this phase may be shortened to only a few months.

Catagen Phase

The catagen phase is relatively short, lasting only 2–3 weeks and involving about 1–2% of scalp hairs at any given time. This duration remains fairly consistent, even in individuals with hair loss conditions. During this phase, the hair follicle undergoes apoptosis, leading to the regression of the lower part of the follicle. The hair bulb detaches from the dermal papilla, and the follicle shrinks. Cellular activity decreases significantly, and the hair shaft becomes club-shaped, preparing for the subsequent telogen phase.

Telogen Phase

In healthy individuals, the telogen phase lasts around 3–4 months and accounts for 10–15% of scalp hairs. However, in those experiencing hair loss, the percentage of hairs in the telogen phase can increase significantly, contributing to noticeable thinning and reduced hair density. During this period, hair growth ceases, and the club hair remains anchored in the follicle. At the end of the telogen phase, the club hair is shed, and the follicle reenters the anagen phase to produce new hair. It is normal for a certain number of hairs to be in the telogen phase at any given time, accounting for the daily shedding of hair.

Factors Influencing Hair Growth

Hair growth and health are influenced by a complex interplay of genetic, hormonal, nutritional, and environmental factors. These factors influence hair growth in a multifaceted manner; there is no one factor that predominates and there is considerable interplay between factors. The precise mechanisms through which these diverse factors culminate in hair growth and loss, and the means through which they may lead to hair loss in one patient while similar conditions may lead to hair retention in another patient are areas of continued investigation.

Genetic Factors

Genes regulate the sensitivity of hair follicles to androgens, which can lead to follicular miniaturization and progressive hair thinning. This genetic predisposition is polygenic, involving multiple genes that influence androgen sensitivity and hair growth cycles. The androgen receptor (AR) gene, located on the X chromosome, plays a crucial role in this process. Variations in the AR gene can increase the sensitivity of hair follicles to androgens, particularly dihydrotestosterone (DHT).

When DHT binds to these hypersensitive androgen receptors in the hair follicles, it triggers a cascade of events that leads to the shortening of the anagen (growth) phase and the prolongation of the telogen (resting) phase of the hair cycle. Over time, this results in the production of progressively shorter, finer hairs—a process known as follicular miniaturization. Eventually, these miniaturized follicles may cease to produce visible hair altogether.

Other genes implicated in androgenetic alopecia include those involved in steroid hormone metabolism (such as SRD5A1 and SRD5A2, which encode 5-α reductase enzymes), growth factor pathways (like the EDA2R gene), and regulators of the hair growth cycle (such as the WNT signaling pathway genes). The complex interplay of these genetic factors determines not only the likelihood of developing androgenetic alopecia but also the pattern, severity, and age of onset of hair loss (Ceruti et al. 2018).

Understanding these genetic mechanisms is crucial for developing targeted therapies and predicting individual responses to treatment. It also explains why androgenetic alopecia often runs in families and why its expression can vary widely among individuals, even within the same family.

Hormonal Influences

Hormones, particularly androgens like testosterone and dihydrotestosterone, as mentioned earlier, have a significant impact on hair growth (Grymowicz 2020). Androgens stimulate hair growth in areas such as the beard and chest while contributing to hair loss on the scalp in genetically predisposed individuals. This regulation of hair growth and loss by continuous exposure to androgens is evident in both the correlation between aging and hair loss, the higher prevalence of androgenetic alopecia in male patients, and the effect of exposure to exogenous androgens and androgen derivatives on hair. The balance of hormones, including estrogen, progesterone, and thyroid hormones, also affects hair growth and health. Aging brings along many hormone imbalances that accelerate hair loss, which is why I always inform my patients that early intervention is crucial for saving the maximum amount of hair (Alonso et al. 2003).

Nutritional Factors

Patients often underestimate the importance of nutrition for the health of hair. Deficiencies in vitamins (e.g., biotin, vitamin D, vitamin E), minerals (e.g., iron, zinc), and proteins can lead to hair loss and poor hair quality. I always remind my patients that factors like nutrition play a pivotal role in hair health. Addressing these factors is essential for effective treatment. A balanced diet rich in essential nutrients, or vitamin supplementation, supports the anagen phase and promotes robust hair growth (Gokce 2022).

1. *Biotin (vitamin B7)*: Supports keratin production and hair growth at doses of 1–5 mg daily, which can be supplemented or consumed through organ meats, fish, eggs, broccoli, and other foods. It is important to note that biotin supplementation can interfere with biotin-based laboratory immunoassays (Patel et al. 2017; Li et al. 2020).
2. *Vitamin D*: Regulates hair follicle cycling and cellular differentiation at doses of 50,000–100,000 IU weekly, which can be supplemented (Sattar et al. 2021; Conic et al. 2021). It is important for practitioners to work with patients to ensure adherence to dosing regimens, as excessive vitamin D consumption can result in toxicity (Galior et al. 2018).
3. *Iron*: Essential for oxygen transport to hair follicles, preventing telogen effluvium. Doses greater than 100 mg daily have been shown to support patient satisfaction in treating telogen effluvium (Soutou et al. 2024).
4. *Zinc*: Crucial for protein synthesis and cell division in hair follicles. Doses of 5 mg/kg/day have been shown to support hair growth in alopecia areata (Berger et al. 2003).

Environmental Factors

External factors such as UV radiation, pollution, chemical exposure, and hair care practices can impact hair health. UV radiation can cause oxidative stress and damage the hair shaft, leading to dryness and brittleness. Pollutants can accumulate on the scalp and hair, interfering with follicular function. Chemical treatments, such as coloring and perming, can weaken hair structure if not performed correctly (Bloch 2019). Proper hair care, including the use of mild shampoos, conditioners, and protective measures, is vital to mitigate these effects.

Shampoos and conditioners are hair care formulations designed to cleanse, protect, and improve the condition of the hair and scalp. Together, shampoos and conditioners protect the hair by maintaining its structural integrity and minimizing environmental damage. Crucial to supporting healthy hair growth is the use of shampoos that cleanse without excessively stripping natural oils, and of conditioners that replenish lost moisture without exposing hair to additional harsh chemicals.

Immune Factors

Recent research has highlighted the significant role of the immune system in hair growth regulation (Rahmani et al. 2020; Wang et al. 2020). The hair follicle has a complex relationship with the immune system, operating under a state of relative immune privilege. Disruptions to this delicate balance can lead to hair loss conditions. For instance, in alopecia areata, T cells attack the hair follicles, leading to patchy hair loss. Conversely, a well-functioning immune system can promote healthy hair growth by regulating inflammation and supporting tissue repair. Cytokines and growth factors produced by immune cells can influence the hair growth cycle, potentially prolonging the anagen phase or triggering premature entry into the catagen phase. Understanding these immune-mediated mechanisms offers new avenues for therapeutic interventions in hair loss disorders.

Clinical Relevance

An in-depth understanding of hair anatomy and physiology is critical for clinicians specializing in hair restoration. This knowledge enables accurate diagnosis of hair loss conditions, development of effective treatment plans, and patient education on maintaining hair health. By comprehending the fundamental aspects of hair growth and the factors influencing it, practitioners can enhance their clinical practice and contribute to advancing hair restoration techniques and therapies.

Chapter 2

Common Causes of Hair Loss

Bilal F. Hamzeh, Julyssa A. Renteria and Robert Dorfman

Introduction

Hair loss, or alopecia, is a complex and multifactorial condition affecting millions of people worldwide. For medical professionals, a thorough understanding of the various causes of hair loss is crucial for accurate diagnosis and effective treatment. This chapter explores the most common causes of hair loss, including androgenetic alopecia, telogen effluvium, and alopecia areata. Additionally, it delves into less common causes such as scarring alopecias, nutritional deficiencies, stress, and various medical conditions (Figure 2.1). By comprehending these diverse etiologies, practitioners can tailor their therapeutic approaches to meet the specific needs of their patients, thereby enhancing treatment efficacy and patient satisfaction.

Androgenetic Alopecia

Androgenetic alopecia (AGA) is a widespread condition, affecting a significant portion of the global population. In men, it impacts approximately 50% by age 50, and up to 80% by age 70.

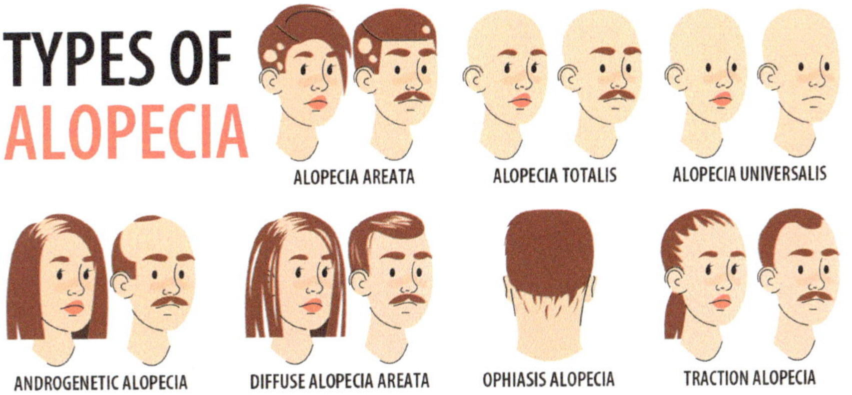

Figure 2.1 Types of alopecia (from Shutterstock, under license).

DOI: 10.1201/9781032726397-2

For women, about 40% experience visible hair loss by age 50. In the United States alone, over 50 million men and 30 million women are affected. These numbers underscore the prevalence of this condition and its far-reaching impact. Importantly, hair loss isn't just a cosmetic issue; it can significantly affect psychological well-being. Studies have shown that hair loss has a profoundly negative effect on the psychological well-being of patients, affecting the self-esteem and social life of as many as 75% of patients (Aukerman and Jaffernay 2023).

AGA is characterized by a progressive thinning of the hair, typically starting at the temples and crown in men and presenting as a general thinning over the entire scalp in women (Oiwoh et al. 2024). The pathophysiology of AGA is rooted in genetic predisposition and hormonal influences. Dihydrotestosterone (DHT), a potent androgen derived from testosterone via the enzyme 5-alpha reductase, plays a central role in the development of AGA. DHT binds to androgen receptors in susceptible hair follicles, leading to follicular miniaturization. Over time, affected hair follicles produce shorter, thinner hairs, eventually leading to the formation of vellus-like, or thin, wispy, "baby" hair and visible thinning.

In men, AGA commonly presents with a receding hairline and balding at the vertex, forming the classic "M" pattern. Women, on the other hand, typically experience diffuse thinning over the crown while preserving the frontal hairline, known as the "Christmas tree" pattern. The diagnosis of AGA is primarily clinical, based on the distinctive pattern of hair loss. Dermoscopic examination can reveal miniaturized hair follicles and increased hair follicle density variation. In some cases, a scalp biopsy may be necessary to confirm the diagnosis and exclude other potential conditions.

See Figures 2.2 and 2.3.

Treatment options for AGA are varied and aim to slow the progression of hair loss and promote hair regrowth (Nestor et al. 2021; Ly et al. 2023). Topical treatments, such as minoxidil and finasteride, are widely used to stimulate hair growth and slow hair loss. Minoxidil works by prolonging the anagen phase of the hair growth cycle and increasing the size of miniaturized hair follicles. Oral medications include minoxidil as well as 5-alpha reductase inhibitors such as finasteride and dutasteride, which reduce DHT levels and are effective in both men and women. For women, spironolactone, an antiandrogen, is often prescribed as well. Spironolactone is a synthetic aldosterone

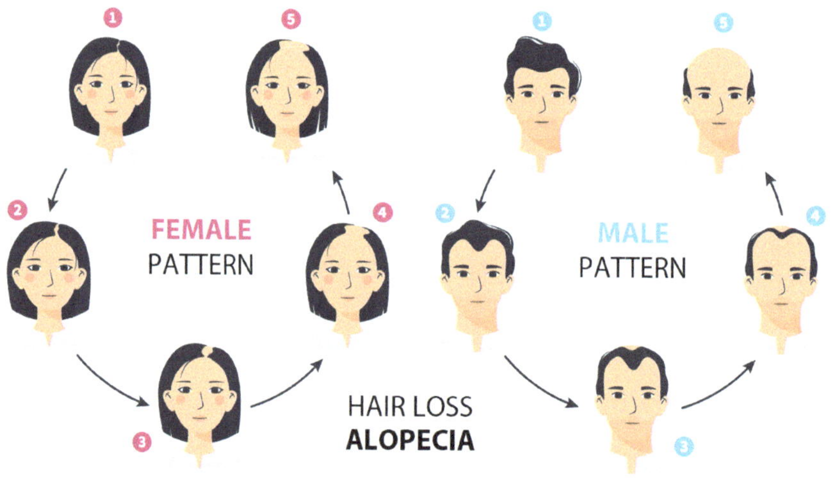

Figure 2.2 Male and female-pattern hair loss (from Shutterstock, under license).

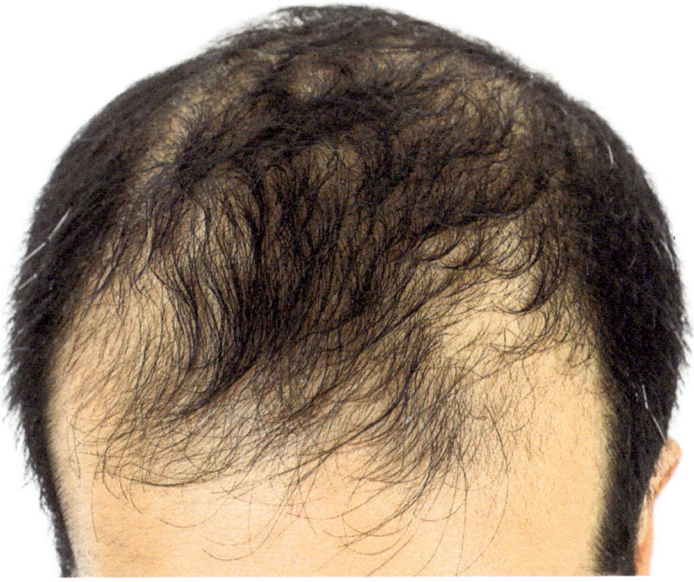

Figure 2.3 Mid-stage male-pattern baldness (from Shutterstock, under license).

antagonist that has been used to treat female-pattern hair loss. It acts both to reduce adrenal synthesis of androgens and as a competitive androgen receptor antagonist, thus mitigating the negative effects of androgens on hair growth. Procedural interventions such as platelet-rich plasma (PRP) therapy, stem cell and exosome therapy, microneedling, low-level laser therapy (LLLT), and laser therapy are emerging treatments with varying degrees of efficacy. PRP therapy involves injecting a concentration of a patient's own platelets into the scalp to stimulate hair growth, while microneedling creates micro-injuries to the scalp to promote healing and hair regrowth. LLLT and laser therapy use specific wavelengths of light to stimulate hair follicles and enhance cellular activity.

Telogen Effluvium

Telogen effluvium (TE) is one of the most common forms of non-scarring alopecia, second only to AGA. While the prevalence is difficult to estimate, telogen effluvium is thought to affect women more than men (Figure 2.4) due to their susceptibility to postpartum hormonal changes (Motosko et al. 2017). The condition can occur at any age but is most frequently observed in adults aged 30–60 years (Whiting 1996).

Notably, TE is often underreported, as many cases resolve spontaneously within 3–6 months. However, chronic TE, lasting more than 6 months, affects about 10% of cases. In terms of hair loss, patients with TE may lose up to 300 hairs per day, compared to the normal 50–100 hairs shed daily in healthy individuals. This dramatic increase in hair shedding can result in a 30–50% reduction in hair volume, which typically diffuses across the scalp.

This condition is often triggered by a physiological or psychological stressor. The pathophysiology of TE involves many hair follicles prematurely entering the telogen phase of the hair growth cycle. Various factors can precipitate this shift, including acute illness, surgery, childbirth,

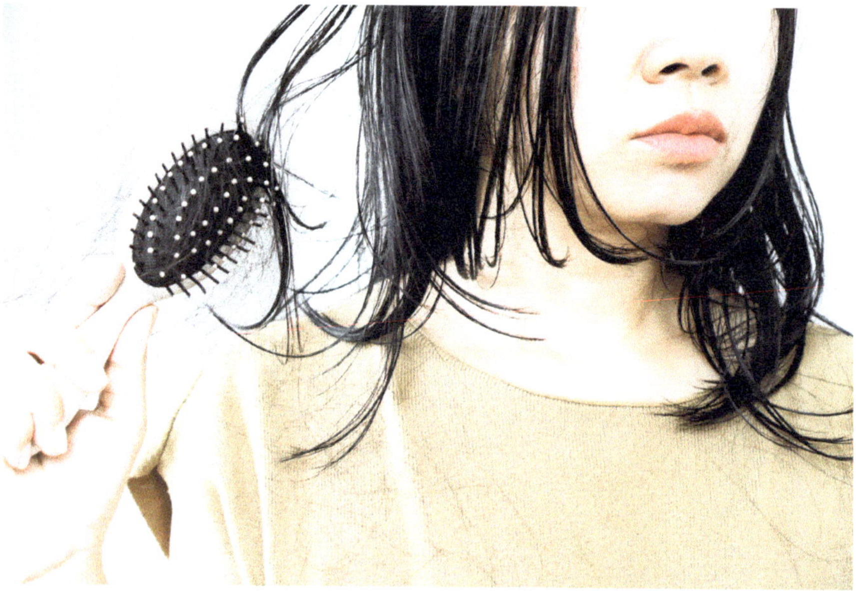

Figure 2.4 **Problem hair in an Asian female (from Shutterstock, under license).**

significant weight loss, and emotional stress (Kligman 1961; Sperling 2001). Nutritional deficiencies and certain medications can also contribute to the development of TE (Harrison and Bergfeld 2009; Rebora 2019).

Common causes of telogen effluvium include:

- Discontinuation of drugs that prolong the anagen phase of hair growth (such as minoxidil or oral contraceptives) (Piraccini et al. 2006).
- Oral retinoids such as acitretin and isotretinoin (Katz et al. 1999; Zhang et al. 2023).
- Fluconazole and other antifungals (Pappas et al. 1995).
- Psychotropic medications including but not limited to valproic acid (Wang et al. 2019), an effect that was found to be dose-dependent (Tomita et al. 2015), lithium carbonate (Malta et al. 2025), and selective serotonin reuptake inhibitors (SSRIs) (Pejcic et al. 2022).
- Anticoagulants such as heparin and warfarin.
- Physiological stress such as recent childbirth or significant weight loss (Chien Yin et al. 2021).
- Infections such as COVID-19 (Sharquie et al. 2022).

Clinically, TE typically presents as diffuse hair thinning without a specific pattern. Patients often report a sudden increase in hair shedding, which is particularly noticeable during washing or brushing their hair. The diagnosis of TE is based on a detailed clinical history and physical examination. A hair pull test, where a small cluster of hairs is gently pulled to see if they come out easily, may be positive, indicating an increased number of telogen hairs. Laboratory tests may be performed to identify any underlying causes, such as thyroid dysfunction or iron deficiency, which can exacerbate hair loss. Dermatoscopy of TE reveals differences when compared with AGA. There is often less hair diameter diversity, and it is typically only seen in frontal areas of the scalp in TE, with fewer yellow/brown dots corresponding to keratin and/or sebum accumulation in the follicular ostia, less vellus hair, and less perifollicular discoloration (Bains et al. 2022). Miniaturization is not seen as often or diffusely in TE as it is in AGA, as most hair follicles are morphologically normal but are in the telogen phase, which is an important distinguishing feature from AGA. Moreover, unlike scarring alopecias, there is no fibrosis and little to no inflammation observed dermoscopically in TE.

Treatment of TE involves addressing the underlying causes (Asghar 2020). This may include treating the underlying medical condition or eliminating the triggering factor. Nutritional support is essential, ensuring adequate intake of essential nutrients such as iron, zinc, and vitamins to support hair regrowth. In some cases, topical treatments like minoxidil may be used to promote hair growth and expedite the resolution of TE. PRP and stem cell/exosome therapy, as well as LLLT and laser therapy, may also be effective in quelling the shedding. One important note regarding telogen effluvium is that most patients recover their normal hair density within 6–9 months after treatment of the underlying cause without much, if any, medical intervention specifically targeted at hair growth (Inamadar 2022). Although TE is distressing for patients, long-term outcomes are among the most favorable when compared with other forms of alopecia because TE is driven by an underlying, often acute and treatable cause. As such, counseling, reassurance, and stress management techniques may also be beneficial for patients experiencing significant psychological stress and are mainstays in the clinical management of TE.

Non-Scarring Alopecia

Alopecia areata (AA) is an autoimmune condition characterized by patchy hair loss on the scalp and other areas of the body (Trüeb and Dias 2018; Figure 2.5). The condition can progress to total scalp hair loss (alopecia totalis; Figure 2.6) or complete body hair loss (alopecia universalis;

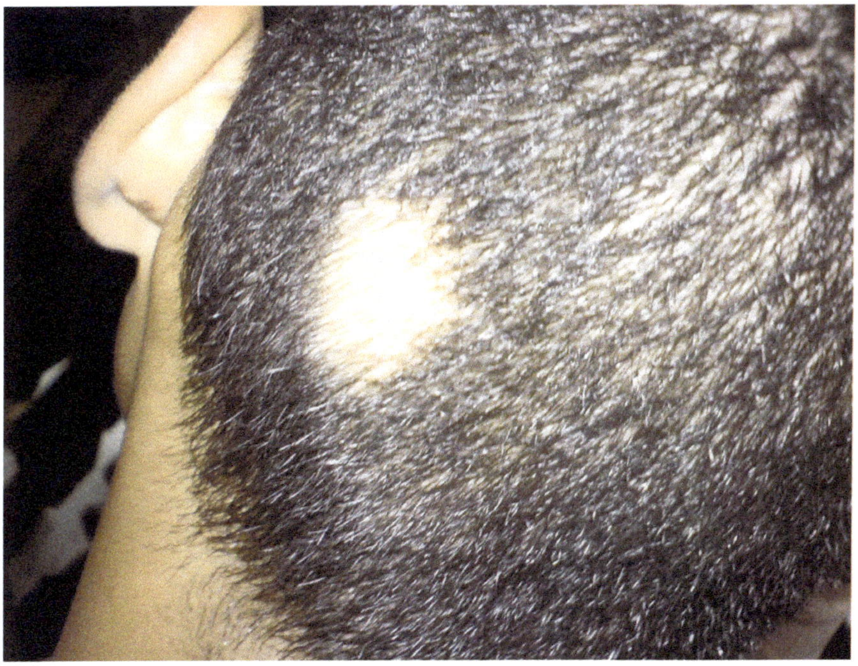

Figure 2.5 **Alopecia areata in a male (from Wikipedia, public domain).**

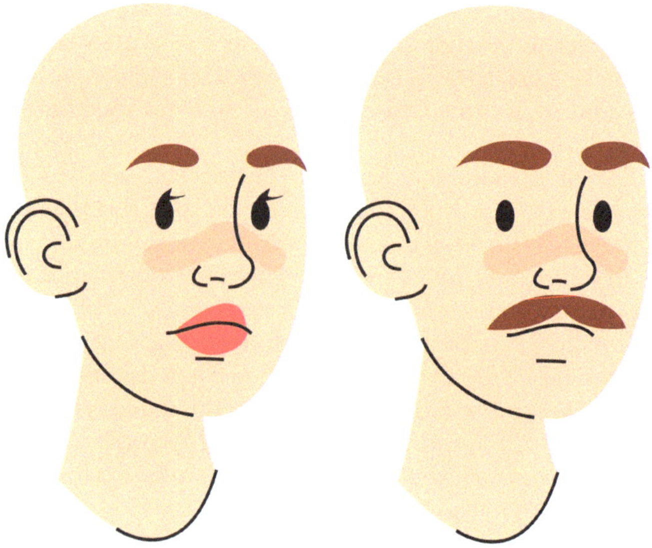

Figure 2.6 Alopecia totalis (from Shutterstock, under license).

Figure 2.7). The pathophysiology of AA involves the immune system mistakenly attacking hair follicles, leading to their premature entry into the telogen phase and subsequent hair loss. Genetic predisposition and environmental factors may contribute to the development of AA.

Clinically, AA presents as well-defined patches of hair loss, which can vary in size and number. Some patients may exhibit nail changes, such as pitting or other nail abnormalities, which can be a helpful diagnostic clue. The ophiasis pattern is a distinct presentation of AA, where hair loss occurs in a band-like pattern around the periphery of the scalp. The diagnosis of AA is primarily clinical, based on the characteristic pattern of hair loss. Dermoscopic examination can show yellow dots, representing inactive follicles with keratin/sebum accumulation, and black dots, representing broken hairs. In atypical cases, a scalp biopsy may be necessary to confirm the diagnosis and exclude other potential conditions. Scalp biopsy in alopecia areata typically reveals numerous polycyclic yellow dots that are diffuse and variable in size and shape, with short, regrowing hairs (Tosti et al. 2008).

Treatment options for AA include topical corticosteroids, which are often the first line of treatment to reduce inflammation and promote hair regrowth. Intralesional corticosteroids, injected directly into the affected areas, can stimulate hair growth and are particularly useful for localized patches (Dahabreh et al. 2023). For less severe cases, PRP, exosome, stem cell, and laser therapies can be tried, along with topical minoxidil applied to the area of hair loss and daily use of LLT. 5-alpha reductase inhibitors are less beneficial in cases of alopecia areata. Topical immunotherapy agents such as diphenylcyclopropenone (DPCP) can induce hair regrowth by modulating the immune response. Systemic treatments, including oral corticosteroids, immunosuppressants, and Janus kinase (JAK) inhibitors, may be used in severe or refractory cases.

JAK inhibitors have shown promise in recent studies, offering a new avenue for treatment in patients with extensive AA (Dillon 2021). Tofacitinib has been shown to be effective in treating AA; one trial demonstrated oral tofacitinib at doses of ≥10 mg daily resulted in ≥90% regrowth

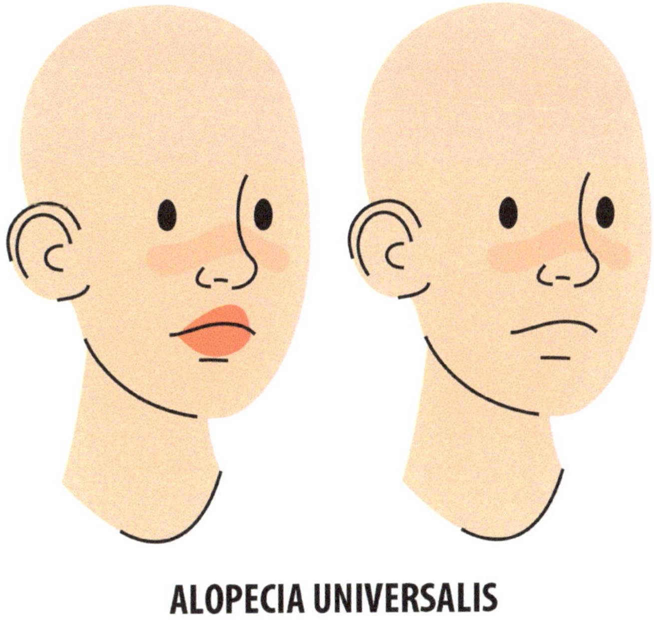

Figure 2.7 **Alopecia universalis (from Shutterstock, under license).**

in patients (Jabbari et al. 2018). Topical tofacitinib has also been evaluated; one study treated patients experiencing AA with 2% topical tofacitinib twice daily and found only 10% of patients experienced significant regrowth (Liu et al. 2018). JAK inhibitors, being more potent and global immunomodulators, are generally reserved only for severe cases of alopecia areata and indeed are only FDA-approved for the management of severe cases. Consideration of the use of JAK inhibitors should be regarded as a last resort after other treatments, such as minoxidil, corticosteroids, PRP/exosomes, and lasers, prove to be ineffective.

There are two JAK inhibitors currently FDA approved for the treatment of severe alopecia areata: baricitinib and ritlecitinib.

Baricitinib (Olumiant)

Baricitinib is an oral, selective, reversible inhibitor of JAK1 and JAK2 and was the first FDA-approved medication for the treatment of AA in 2022, with 2 or 4 mg doses indicated to be taken once daily (orally) for AA. Other indications for the use of baricitinib include rheumatoid arthritis and treatment of COVID-19 (Gupta et al. 2022). Phase 3 clinical trials showed a significant improvement in patients experiencing AA following treatment with baricitinib compared with placebo. Side effects in the treatment group included acne, elevated creatine kinase levels, and elevated HDL and LDL cholesterol levels (King et al. 2022). Other side effects included headaches, upper respiratory tract and urinary tract infections, and nasopharyngitis. Patients continued to show improvement in hair growth beyond week 52, including growth of the eyelashes and eyebrows, indicating potential for long-term efficacy of the treatment (Senna et al. 2024).

Ritlecitinib (Litfulo)

Ritlecitinib is an oral, irreversible inhibitor of JAK3 and the TEC kinase family, the second of its class to be approved for use in the treatment of AA in 2023 at doses of 30 or 50 mg taken orally once daily. A phase 3 clinical trial showed ritlecitinib to be an effective and well-tolerated treatment in adolescent and adult alopecia areata, demonstrating hair growth including growth of the eyelashes and eyebrows with few treatment-limiting side effects that included headache, acne, increased risk for infections, and nasopharyngitis, similar to baricitinib (King et al. 2023).

Scarring Alopecias

Scarring alopecias differ in their clinical presentation, management, and histological manifestation compared to non-scarring alopecias. Unlike the non-scarring alopecias described earlier, scarring alopecias result in permanent loss of hair follicles, replacing them with scar tissue. While non-scarring alopecias preserve the potential for hair regrowth, resulting in a quiescence of the hair follicle, scarring alopecias result in complete loss of the hair follicle with little to no potential for regrowth. Examples of scarring alopecias include central centrifugal cicatricial alopecia (CCCA), discoid lupus erythematosus (DLE), and lichen planopilaris (LPP).

The diagnostic differentiation between scarring and non-scarring alopecias is crucial because of the differences in management between the groups of hair loss disorders. Notably, patients experiencing scarring alopecias cannot undergo hair transplantation due to the nature of follicle fibrosis in these conditions, making scalp biopsies an essential step before proceeding to transplantation if there is any ambiguity regarding the etiology of the hair loss.

Central Centrifugal Cicatricial Alopecia (CCCA)

CCCA is one type of scarring alopecia that results in permanent loss of hair, typically presenting with small, round patches of hair loss around the center of the scalp that spread centrifugally. CCCA can also present with inflammation and small, raised bumps on the scalp, although many patients are asymptomatic (Callender et al. 2012). It most commonly affects women of African descent with prevalence ranging from 2.7% to 5.7%, but it can affect anyone (Dlova et al. 2017). CCCA can be diagnosed via non-invasive dermoscopy, which can show a perihilar white/gray halo, corresponding to fibrotic lesions of melanocytes (Herskovitz and Miteva, 2016). As CCCA is a scarring alopecia, the onset of disease is associated with inflammation, which can be appreciated on biopsy and corresponds to the progression of disease. The additional symptoms that CCCA can present with occur secondary to this inflammation, which eventually leads to fibrosis of hair follicles. Treatment and progression of CCCA depend on the presence or lack of inflammation, indicating whether there is stabilization. See Figures 2.8 and 2.9.

Discoid Lupus Erythematosus (DLE)

DLE is a scarring alopecia that is a variant of chronic lupus erythematosus (CLE), a chronic autoimmune condition mediated by the deposition of immune complexes and subsequent plaque and scar formation (Figure 2.10). DLE presents initially with non-scarring scaly and erythematosus papules. These papules result from underlying autoimmune processes and can lead to hyper- and hypopigmentation and eventually progress to form plaques with variable presentation that can be

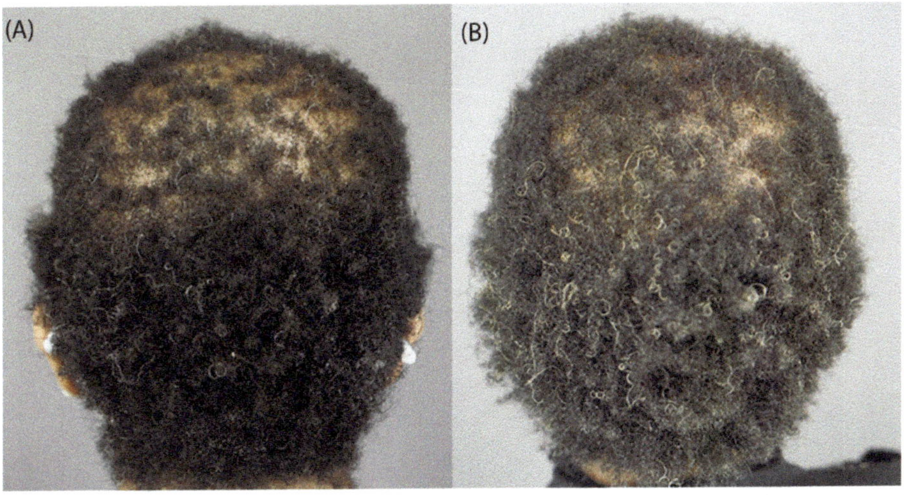

Figure 2.8 **(A) Vertex and posterior scalp of a patient with central centrifugal cicatricial alopecia obtained 13 months after micronized fat injection, oral minoxidil, topical Gashee applications (once daily), and oral Gashee supplements. (B) Images of the same area 3 months after the treatment changed to topical Gashee treatments (twice daily) and oral minoxidil. (From S Umar et al., Treatment-refractory central centrifugal cicatricial alopecia responsive to a novel botanical treatment, *Clin Cosmet Investig Dermatol.* 2022;15:609–619, with permission).**

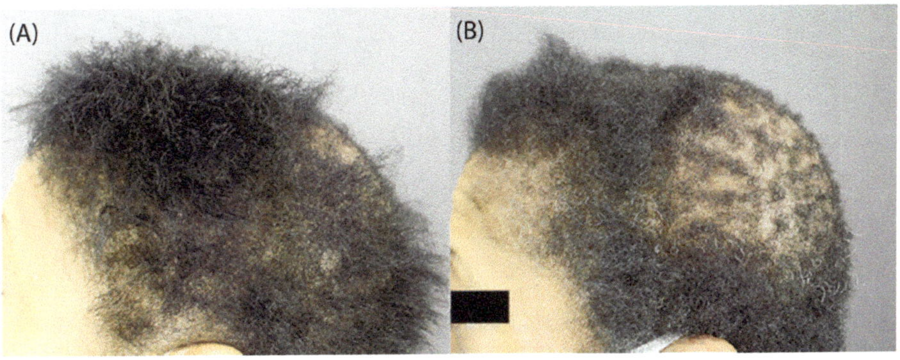

Figure 2.9 **Left parietal area and vertex of a patient diagnosed with central centrifugal cicatricial alopecia obtained before (A) and after (B) 5 months of treatment with topical Gashee (applied once daily), and two sessions of platelet-rich plasma scalp injections are shown. (From S Umar et al., Treatment-refractory central centrifugal cicatricial alopecia responsive to a novel botanical treatment. *Clin Cosmet Investig Dermatol.* 2022;15:609–619, with permission).**

accompanied by fibrosis and atrophy. Lesions can be pruritic, tender, or otherwise asymptomatic (Concha and Werth, 2018).

DLE has a higher incidence in racial minorities, specifically in patients of African descent. Moreover, these patients often present with worse baseline scores (Cutaneous Lupus Erythematosus Disease Area and Severity Index [CLASI]) (Joseph et al. 2021). As such, DLE is most prevalent in Black women, presenting most often in early to middle adulthood. Newer studies have conversely shown that although DLE is more prevalent in Black populations, race was not significantly

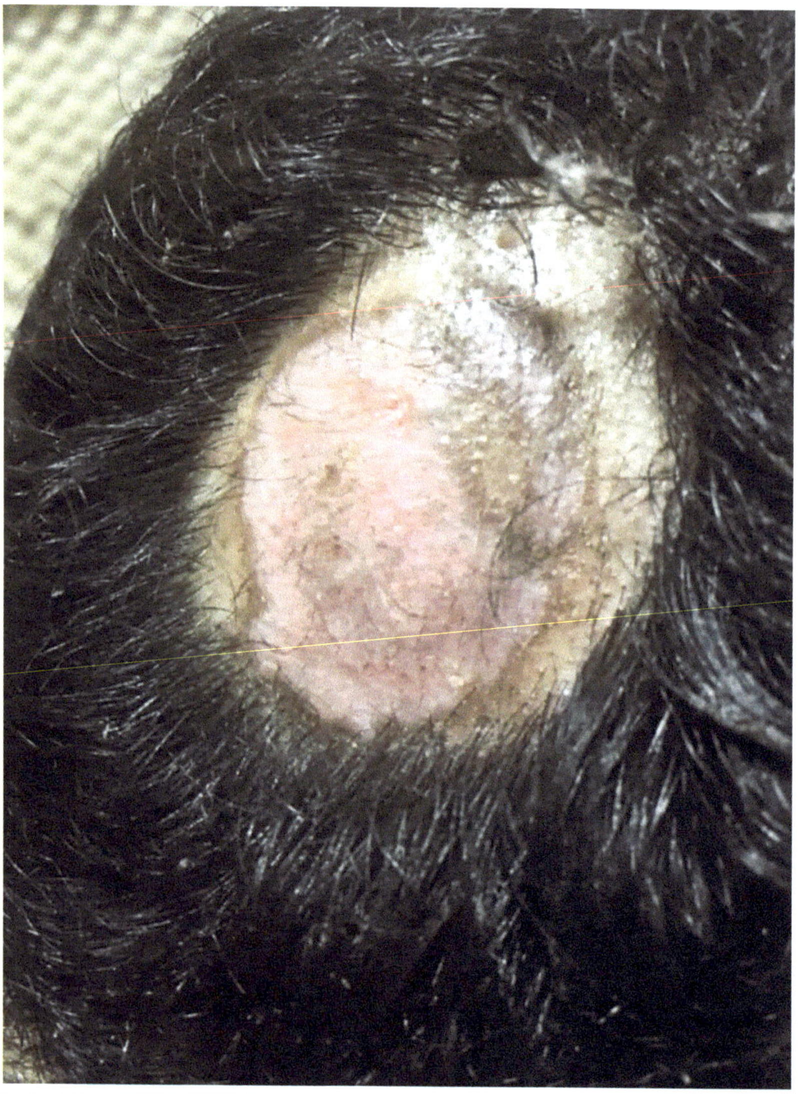

Figure 2.10 Discoid lupus erythematosus (from Mohammed 2018/Wikipedia, under Creative Commons Attribution).

associated with disease severity; however, other factors such as smoking status did have an association with more severe damage (Faden et al. 2024).

DLE is often diagnosed histologically and via trichoscopy (Desai and Miteva 2021). Histologically, DLE shows a lymphocytic infiltrate consistent with autoimmune mediation of the disease process, basement membrane thickening, reduced sebaceous glands, follicular hyperkeratosis, and pan-follicular inflammation that can eventually lead to follicle atrophy and fibrosis (Chung and Goldberg 2017). Trichoscopy shows arborizing vessels, follicular keratotic plugs, and red dots in addition to peripilar scale and erythema (Żychowska and Żychowska 2021).

Lichen Planopilaris (LPP)

LPP, a form of lichen planus that affects the skin, nails, hair, and mucous membranes, is very similar in etiology and presentation to DLE, being mediated by an underlying autoimmune process and preferentially affecting the mucous membranes, skin, hair, and nails. LPP is not caused by lichen; rather, it is named for the lichen-like appearance of the associated lesions. Like DLE, LPP presents clinically with patchy and progressive lesions, often purple plaques that affect the center of the scalp and can extend beyond the scalp to affect other hair-bearing regions of the body (Lepe et al. 2024). LPP can also present with irritation, including itching, scaling, burning, and tenderness of affected regions, in addition to increased hair shedding (Kang et al. 2008). LPP most frequently affects older women, most often postmenopausal women taking hormonal therapies (Meinhard et al. 2014). See Figures 2.11 and 2.12.

Histologically, LPP presents with arborizing vessels, peripilar tubular casts, and erythema consistent with early stages. Blue-gray and irregular white fibrotic dots, in addition to milky red areas observed in a "target" pattern via dermoscopy, are consistent with later stages of LPP (Gowda et al. 2024; Ankad et al. 2013).

Tinea Capitis

Tinea capitis is a highly contagious superficial scalp infection that most commonly infects children, with the peak incidence between 3 to 7 years of age, generally affecting men and women equally, although it is not frequently seen in adults (Figures 2.13 and 2.14). The most common predisposing factors for tinea capitis in adults include immunosuppression, resulting from conditions such as HIV/AIDS or other immunosuppressive syndromes or from long-standing use of corticosteroids, diabetes, contact with animals, and infections present elsewhere on the body (Dhurat et al. 2021). Infection can also occur as a result of changes in scalp conditions, such as changes in pH and fatty acid composition of sebum caused by hormonal changes such as menopause in women (Salazar et al. 2018). Outside of these predisposing risk factors, poor scalp hygiene and communal sharing of hair care tools, in addition to frequent head wrapping, can increase the risk of developing tinea capitis due to changes in scalp conditions and repeated exposure to the fungal organisms that cause infection (Takwale et al. 2001). Tinea capitis infection is most commonly caused by the organisms *Trichophyton tonsurans* and *Microsporum canis*, and can present as either inflammatory or non-inflammatory.

Diagnosis

Non-inflammatory tinea capitis infection can present in a seborrheic form with scaling but void of significant hair loss, or fine scaling with circular patches of alopecia; adherent, sometimes pustular scaling on the scalp that can mimic dandruff, either diffuse or localized; and/or the appearance of black dots in addition to corkscrew, zigzag, and comma hair representing structural damage and broken hairs (Leung et al. 2020). Comma hair, corkscrew hair, and pigtail hairs have been described as distinguishing features in tinea capitis (Slowinska et al. 2008; El-Taweel et al. 2014), each representing disintegration, cracking, and bending due to the presence of fungal hyphae within the hair shaft (Elghblawi et al. 2016). Inflammatory tinea capitis can include all of these features in addition to keroins, which are inflammatory masses (Pomeranz and Sabnis 2002). In children, tinea capitis can often be easier to diagnose, presenting with pruritus, scaling, and

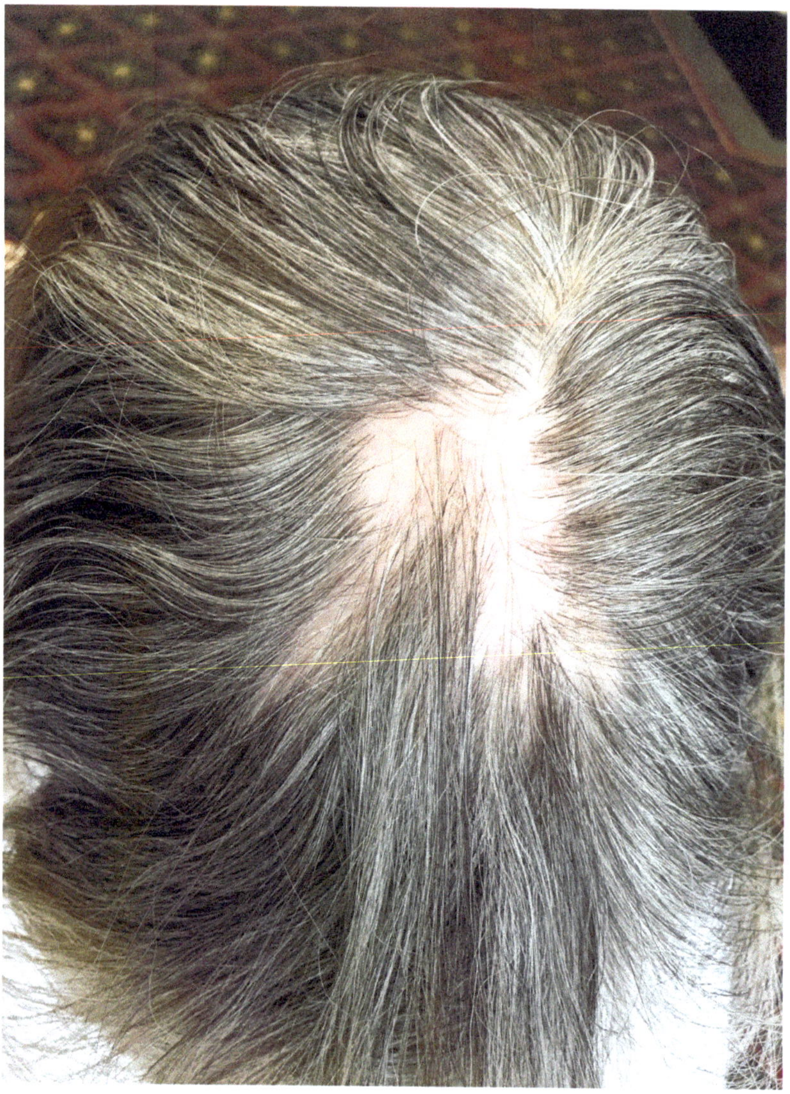

Figure 2.11 **Scarring alopecia (from Scarring Alopecia Foundation, with permission).**

lymphadenopathy in addition to hair loss. In adults, infection can be more subtle, variable, and is often void of other symptoms, requiring a high index of suspicion and exclusion of other possible etiologies to diagnose (Salazar et al. 2018).

Scalp biopsy often reveals no evidence of fibrosis, with minimal inflammatory perifollicular inflammatory infiltrate observed. Although potassium hydroxide (KOH) observation, a microscopic technique that involves application of KOH to scalp biopsies to reveal fungal elements, and fungal culture have historically been considered the gold standard in the diagnosis of tinea capitis, the time-consuming nature and high rate of false negatives associated with these procedures may make trichoscopy an improved principal mode of diagnosis for tinea capitis. Culture, microscopy including KOH microscopy, or fungus-specific staining, such as Sabouraud's dextrose agar or

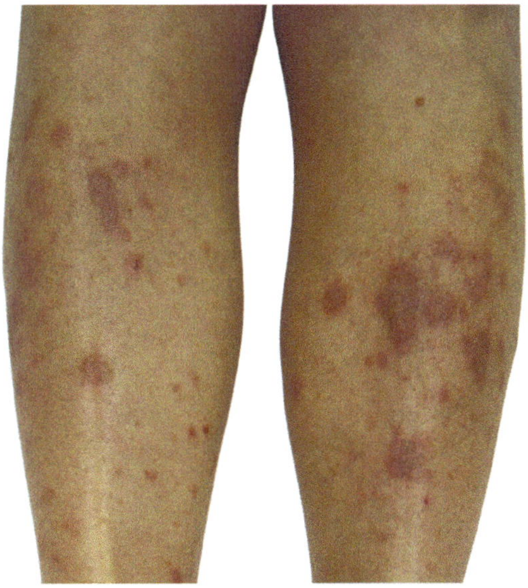

Figure 2.12 Lichen planus affecting the legs (from Shutterstock, under license).

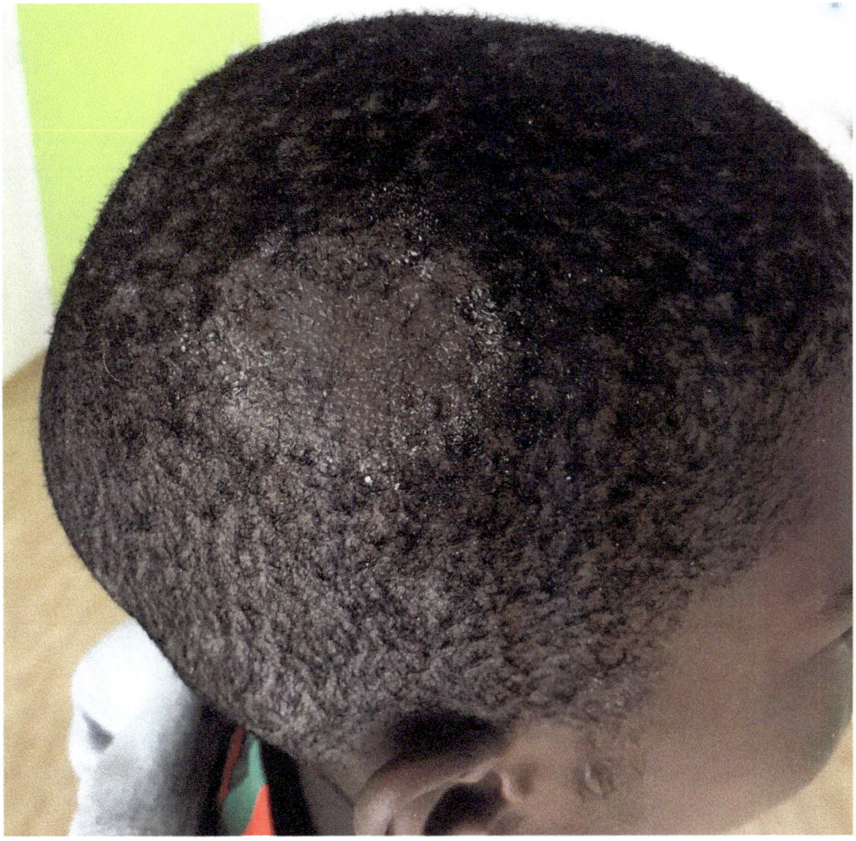

Figure 2.13 Tinea capitis (from Gzzz/Wikipedia, under Creative Commons Attribution license).

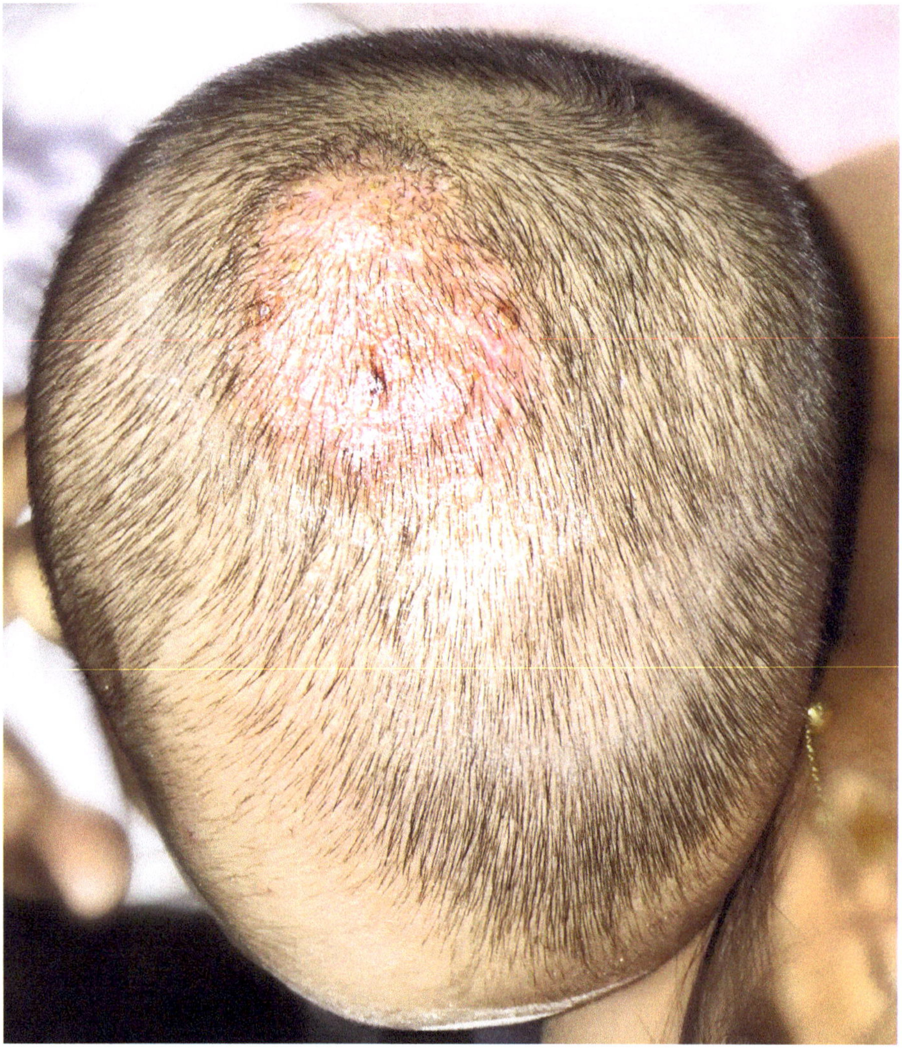

Figure 2.14 **Tinea capitis (from Shutterstock, under license).**

Chicago blue staining, are useful diagnostic tools but do, as mentioned, have a high rate of false negatives (Hubbard 1999).

Treatment

The antifungal medication griseofulvin has historically been the first-line treatment of tinea capitis (Bennett et al. 2000), however the long treatment courses, often ranging from 6 to 8 weeks of oral dosing, and the risks for hepatotoxicity at the required doses, particularly in children, in addition to treatment failure rates that can be as high as 39.3%, have led practitioners to favor other potential treatments (Blumer 1999; Abdel Rahman et al. 1997). Terbinafine, another antifungal, has been preferred in the treatment for tinea capitis, demonstrating a higher complete cure rate than griseofulvin in some studies (Gupta et al. 2018), with clinical trials demonstrating that a 4-week course of once-daily oral dosing is required in the treatment of tinea capitis, much shorter than is often indicated when prescribing griseofulvin (Tey et al. 2011). Some studies have even found 2-week courses of terbinafine to be effective in the treatment of certain causes of tinea capitis, specifically caused by *Trichophyton* species of fungi (Friedlander et al. 2002; Haroon et al. 1996). However, the question of whether griseofulvin, terbinafine, or other antifungals are most effective in the treatment of tinea capitis has been shown to be most dependent on the causative organism, with some medications being more effective in the treatment of tinea capitis caused by certain species of fungi than others (Gupta et al. 2013).

Itraconazole, an azole-class antifungal, has also been shown to be effective in the treatment of tinea capitis depending on the causative organism; however, it is not FDA approved for tinea capitis in the United States despite being among the most popular treatments in many European countries (Fuller et al. 2014), demonstrating efficacy in the treatment of *Trichophyton* infections that is similar to that observed with oral terbinafine (Gupta et al. 2001). Ketoconazole, a well-tolerated azole-class antifungal with antiandrogenic properties, is frequently used for dandruff and hair loss, and may be an effective first-line or adjunctive treatment in tinea capitis, often posing a reduced risk of side effects due to topical administration of the drug (Greer 2000), although some studies have demonstrated inferior efficacy of oral ketoconazole relative to oral griseofulvin (Tanz et al. 1988). Topical selenium sulfide, another over-the-counter antifungal, has also been shown to be an effective adjunct in the treatment of tinea capitis, posing an additional potential benefit of reducing the spread of spores to others (Allen et al. 1982). Fluconazole is similar to itraconazole, but has been shown to be inferior to other treatments in some studies such as that conducted by Gupta et al. in 2001, while other studies have shown it to be superior to griseofulvin in the treatment of pediatric tinea capitis (Foster et al. 2005). This variability can, again, likely be attributed to differences in the causative organisms between patients.

Systemic antifungal therapies all have similar side effects ranging from nausea, pruritus, headache, vomiting, mild abdominal discomfort, and GI upset to liver toxicity, elevated serum triglycerides, elevated serum uric acid, anemia, eosinophilia, leukocytosis and granulocytopenia (Memisoglu et al. 1999; Haroon et al. 1995). Lab monitoring is not typically required for the course durations indicated for the treatment of tinea capitis with most agents, but preexisting liver disease or clinical suspicion of liver injury, hematological, or metabolic side effects may require routine monitoring of LFTs, triglycerides, and WBC counts.

Nutritional Deficiencies

Nutritional deficiencies can significantly impact hair health and lead to diffuse hair loss (Almohanna et al. 2019). Common deficiencies include iron, zinc, biotin, and vitamin D. Iron deficiency, particularly prevalent in premenopausal women, is a well-known cause of hair loss. Iron is essential for oxygen transport to hair follicles, and its deficiency can lead to telogen effluvium. Zinc plays a crucial role in protein synthesis and cell division in hair follicles, and its deficiency can impair hair growth and lead to hair thinning. Biotin, also known as vitamin B7, supports keratin production and hair growth, and its deficiency can result in hair thinning and brittle nails. Vitamin D is involved in hair follicle cycling and immune regulation, and its deficiency can contribute to hair loss.

The management of hair loss due to nutritional deficiencies involves correcting the deficiency through dietary modifications and supplementation. Ensuring an adequate intake of essential nutrients can support hair regrowth and improve overall hair health. A balanced diet rich in vitamins, minerals, and proteins is vital for maintaining healthy hair growth.

Stress

Psychological stress can trigger telogen effluvium and exacerbate other forms of hair loss. Chronic stress can disrupt the hair growth cycle, leading to increased shedding and thinning (Thom 2016). The exact mechanism by which stress affects hair growth is not fully understood, but it is believed that stress hormones such as cortisol may play a role. High levels of cortisol can affect the hair follicles, pushing them into the telogen phase prematurely.

Managing stress is an essential component of treating stress-related hair loss. This may involve stress management techniques such as mindfulness, meditation, and cognitive-behavioral therapy. In some cases, pharmacological interventions may be necessary to manage severe stress or anxiety.

Medical Conditions

Various medical conditions can contribute to hair loss, including thyroid disorders, autoimmune diseases, and infections. Hypothyroidism and hyperthyroidism can both cause diffuse hair thinning. Thyroid hormones play a crucial role in regulating the hair growth cycle, and imbalances can disrupt this process (Cohen et al. 2023). Autoimmune diseases such as lupus (Udompanich et al. 2018) and rheumatoid arthritis can affect hair growth, either directly by attacking hair follicles or indirectly through systemic inflammation and the use of immunosuppressive medications.

The management of hair loss due to medical conditions involves treating the underlying condition. For thyroid disorders, this may include hormone replacement therapy or antithyroid medications. For autoimmune diseases, immunosuppressive therapies may be necessary to control the disease and reduce inflammation. Antifungal treatments are used to treat scalp infections and restore hair growth (Nestor 2021).

Drug-Induced Alopecia

Drug-induced alopecia occurs when certain medications (Table 2.1) interfere with the normal hair growth cycle, leading to hair loss. This condition is typically a form of telogen effluvium, where hair prematurely enters the resting (telogen) phase, resulting in diffuse shedding several weeks to months after starting the medication. Some drugs, however, may cause anagen effluvium, where hair falls out during the active growth phase. Common culprits include chemotherapy agents, which rapidly damage dividing hair follicle cells, as well as beta-blockers, antidepressants, anticoagulants, and retinoids (Chon et al. 2012). The severity of hair loss can vary depending on the drug and individual response, and in most cases, hair regrowth resumes once the offending medication is discontinued or the body adjusts to it. Identifying drug-induced alopecia early is critical for reversing the condition and managing patient concerns. Common agents known to induce hair loss are also discussed in the section "Telogen Effluvium."

Table 2.1 Drug-Induced Alopecia

Drugs That Can Cause Telogen Effluvium
Heparin
Warfarin
Propranolol/metoprolol
Captopril/enalapril
Allopurinol
Boric acid
Phenytoin
Glibenclamide
Amphetamines
Levadopa
Bromocryptine
Methysergide
Interferon
Albendazole/mebendazole
Cimetidine
Colchicine (low dose)
Sulfasalazine
Penicillamine
Gold
Drugs with Anti-Thyroid Action
Carbimazole
Propylthiouracil
Amiodorone
Lithium
Drugs with Anti-Hyperlipidemic Action
Clofibrate
Triparanol
Drugs with Pro-Androgen Action
Oral contraceptive pill
Danazol
Testosterone
Anabolic steroids
Chemotherapeutics

Source: From Sinclair and Dawber (2001), with permission.

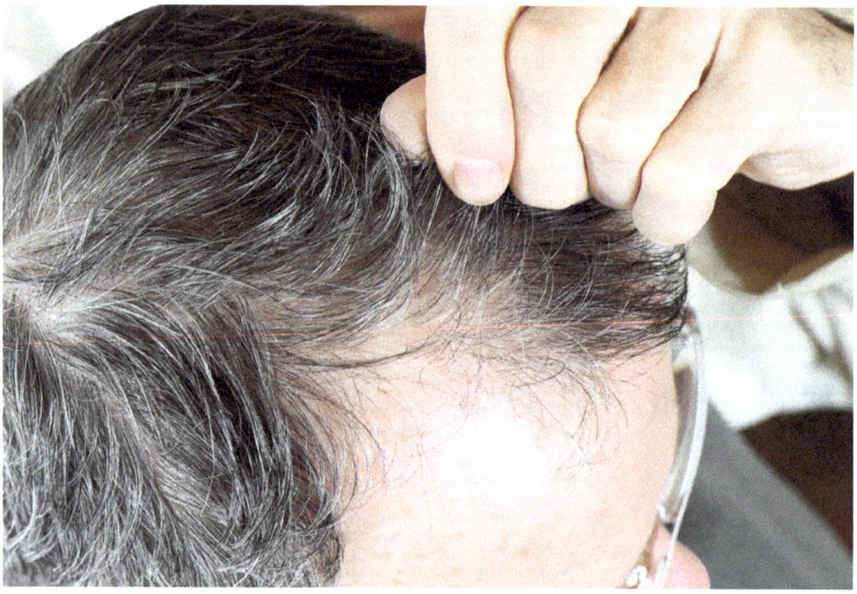

Figure 2.15 **Trichotillomania (from Shutterstock, under license).**

Trichotillomania

Trichotillomania, or hair-pulling disorder, is a psychological condition characterized by repetitive and compulsive pulling of one's hair, often leading to functional impairment, loss of hair density, and distress (Figure 2.15). Trichotillomania has been identified in as much as 1.7% of the population, with one study finding no significant difference in prevalence between men and women and an average age of onset of 17.7 years. The condition often coincides with other psychiatric comorbidities such as generalized anxiety disorder (GAD), obsessive–compulsive disorder (OCD), post-traumatic stress disorder (PTSD), and attention-deficit hyperactivity disorder (ADHD) (Grant et al. 2020). The *Diagnostic and Statistical Manual of Mental Disorders*, 5th edition (*DSM-5*) describes trichotillomania under OCD and related conditions, alongside skin picking disorder (excoriation), body dysmorphic disorder (BDD), and hoarding disorder (American Psychiatric Association 2013).

Trichotillomania is diagnosed clinically via patient interview; practitioners can ask patients questions pertaining to any hair pulling behaviors including habitually combing through the hair, twirling strands of hair, or directly removing hair. Published interviews, such as the Trichotillomania Diagnostic Interview, can be utilized or adapted by practitioners for this purpose (Rothbaum and Ninan 1994). Other standardized clinical assessments, such as the NIMH Trichotillomania Severity Scale (NIMH-TSS) and the NIMH Trichotillomania Impairment Scale (NIMH-TIS), are other standardized questionnaires that can be employed by practitioners to aid in the clinical diagnosis of the condition (Diefenbach 2005).

Direct measures of hair loss due to trichotillomania should also be utilized in the clinical diagnosis of the condition, utilizing photograph ratings, bald spot measurements, and collected pulled hair. Focal losses of hair that are not characteristic of typical female-pattern hair loss or male-pattern hair loss that are void of lesions can raise clinical suspicion for trichotillomania and warrant further investigation. Hair pulling results in irregularly shaped patchy hair loss with broken hairs of varying lengths, and can lead to scarring from repetitive stress and removal (Mostaghimi 2012).

Upon diagnosis of trichotillomania, practitioners should refer patients to licensed psychiatrists for further evaluation and management, often involving a combination of talk therapy and medication management, which often mirrors the clinical management of obsessive–compulsive disorder.

Traction Alopecia

Traction alopecia is a form of hair loss that results from chronic pulling forces on hair roots, often occurring as a result of hair styling and/or hair type. Traction alopecia is thus commonly seen in the hair of women of Afro-Caribbean descent, often having tight and curly or spiraling hair, and in women who wear their hair in tight braids, ponytails, attach weaves or hair extensions, or wear other styles that result in a chronic pulling force on hair roots (Figure 2.16). For these reasons, traction alopecia is seen much more commonly in women than in men, and much more commonly in women of Afro-Caribbean descent, although it can affect anyone (Khumalo 2012). Another distinct cause of traction alopecia is the chemical relaxation of the hair in which hair is treated to disrupt the disulfide linkages that produce curling or spiraling of the hair in an effort to straighten hair (Khumalo et al. 2007).

It can affect up to one-third of women of African descent at some point in their lives and has a biphasic clinical progression in which early stages are marked by reversible loss of hair shafts due to traction, while later stages are characterized by scarring and irreversible scarring alopecia due to chronic trauma to hair roots (Billero and Miteva 2018). During the early clinical stages, often appreciated in childhood, non-scarring hair loss can be observed in the areas experiencing tension.

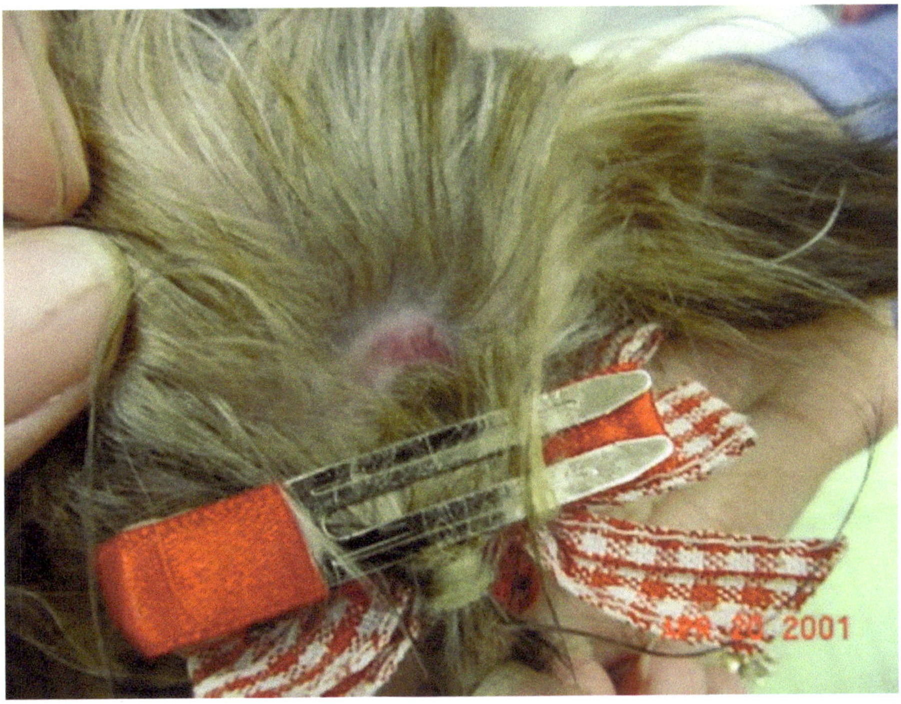

Figure 2.16 Traction alopecia (from Wikipedia, under Creative Commons Attribution license).

Hair loss can resemble an ophiasis or snake-like pattern, showing broken hair of varying lengths, similar to trichotillomania, perifollicular erythema, and intrafollicular pustules microscopically (Heath and Taylor 2012). Later stages are marked by an irreversible scarring alopecia characterized by the replacement of terminal hair follicles with fibrotic fibrous tracts, with preservation of sebaceous glands and no perifollicular inflammatory cells, and can be accompanied by tenderness, itching, paresthesias, and headaches (Hwang et al. 1999).

Treatment of traction alopecia depends on the stage of progression. Initial management of non-scarring traction alopecia includes addressing the underlying cause and avoiding chemical treatment and trauma to the hair. Counseling patients on proper hair treatment and potential sources of trauma that contribute to traction alopecia is crucial. Combating the inflammation that characterizes this initial stage is often accomplished with topical or oral corticosteroids and/or topical or oral antibiotics with anti-inflammatory properties (Lawson et al. 2017). One study published in 2007 described the case of two women who had experienced no regrowth after two years of abstention from traumatic hairstyling practices, but experienced significant regrowth with the administration of 2% topical minoxidil after 6 months (Khumalo and Ngwanya 2007). Late-stage or scarring traction alopecia is more difficult to treat, with some studies showing surgical hair transplantation as being a potentially viable option (Earles 1986).

Clinical Relevance

Understanding the diverse causes of hair loss is essential for accurate diagnosis and effective treatment. Medical professionals must consider multiple factors, including genetic predisposition, hormonal influences, nutritional status, psychological health, and underlying medical conditions when evaluating and managing patients with hair loss. This comprehensive approach enables the development of personalized treatment plans that address the unique needs of each patient, enhancing therapeutic outcomes and patient satisfaction.

By integrating this knowledge into clinical practice, practitioners can improve their diagnostic accuracy and therapeutic strategies. An in-depth understanding of hair anatomy, physiology, and the factors influencing hair growth allows clinicians to develop effective treatment plans and educate patients on maintaining hair health. This knowledge also supports the advancement of hair restoration techniques and therapies, contributing to the overall improvement of patient care in the field of hair loss and restoration.

Chapter 3

Female-Pattern Hair Loss

Haley Guinan and Robert Dorfman

Introduction

Female-pattern hair loss (FPHL) presents unique challenges distinct from male-pattern baldness. Women typically experience a diffuse thinning across the mid-frontal scalp with preservation of the frontal hairline, whereas men show more concentrated recession at the temples and vertex. Complete baldness is rare in women– most affected females report a gradual reduction in density rather than total loss. Because female hair loss is often less severe and more diffuse, women are generally more inclined to seek non-surgical treatments (e.g., topical or hormonal therapies) rather than hair transplant surgery. This growing demand for non-invasive solutions underscores the need for a nuanced approach tailored to the specific etiologies, patterns, and psychosocial impacts of hair loss in women. Notably, FPHL can have a significant psychosocial impact, with studies showing impaired quality of life and higher rates of anxiety or depression proportional to the severity of hair loss (Hwang et al. 2024). Effective management therefore requires both medical and supportive strategies.

Hormonal Influences on Female-Pattern Hair Loss

Androgens play a central role in male androgenetic alopecia, but their influence in female-pattern hair loss is more complex. Females produce lower levels of the potent androgens, testosterone and dihydrotestosterone (DHT) compared to males, which partly explains the different pattern of thinning. In men, high local DHT levels trigger follicular miniaturization in androgen-sensitive regions, producing defined bald patches. In women, the lower androgen levels and possibly differing follicular sensitivity lead to a more diffuse thinning without overt bald patches (Fabbrocini et al. 2018). In fact, FPHL may even develop in some women without any abnormal elevation in circulating androgens (Herskovitz and Tosti 2013). This suggests that while androgens (particularly DHT) are important – binding to androgen receptors in hair follicle dermal papilla cells to shorten the growth (anagen) phase—other factors are also at play (Martinez-Jacobo et al. 2018). These hormonal variations in testosterone and DHT between men and women influence their respective hair loss patterns. Males typically exhibit concentrated thinning at the temples and crown, creating a clearly defined baldness pattern. In contrast, females generally experience diffuse

DOI: 10.1201/9781032726397-3

thinning across the mid-frontal scalp, with preservation of the frontal hairline. Complete baldness in women is rare; instead, they commonly report a gradual reduction in overall hair density. This difference primarily stems from comparatively lower androgen levels—specifically testosterone and DHT—in females, hormones that, as discussed in Chapter 1, are principally responsible for hair follicle miniaturization (Fabbrocini et al. 2018). (Fabbrocini et al. 2018).

One key hormone difference is that estrogens appear to have a protective effect on hair follicles. Estrogen can prolong the anagen phase of the hair cycle and promote hair growth by enhancing growth factor production in the follicle (Rinaldi et al. 2023). It also has vasodilatory effects that improve scalp blood flow, ensuring oxygen and nutrient delivery to follicles (Rinaldi et al. 2023). This may explain why women often notice fuller, thicker hair during high-estrogen states (for example, pregnancy) and why hair thinning often accelerates when estrogen levels fall (as in postpartum or menopause). Conversely, conditions that increase androgen activity or reduce estrogen influence can exacerbate FPHL. For instance, women with hyperandrogenic conditions like polycystic ovary syndrome (PCOS) sometimes develop female-pattern thinning or even male-pattern hair loss due to increased local DHT effects (Brough and Torgerson 2017). Similarly, the androgen-to-estrogen ratio rises during menopause as estrogen declines, allowing androgens to exert a relatively greater influence on hair follicles. We discuss these life-stage hormonal fluctuations in more detail later, as they critically shape the onset and progression of FPHL in women.

Pathophysiology of Female-Pattern Hair Loss

The pathophysiology of FPHL is polygenic and multifactorial, involving a complex interplay of genetic predisposition, hormonal factors, and environmental influences. Although FPHL and male-pattern hair loss share the final common pathway of progressive follicular miniaturization, emerging evidence suggests the underlying causes are not identical in the two sexes (Fabbrocini et al. 2018). Genetic studies have identified several candidate loci for susceptibility. Notably, variants in the androgen receptor (AR) gene on the X-chromosome have been linked to male balding and may also contribute to FPHL by increasing follicular sensitivity to normal androgen levels (Fabbrocini et al. 2018). This means a genetically predisposed woman might experience follicle miniaturization even with circulating androgens in the normal female range. Two large genome-wide association studies found over 60 genetic loci associated with male androgenetic alopecia, many of which are thought to overlap with female hair loss genetics (Heilmann-Heimbach et al. 2017) (Pickrell et al. 2016). However, when investigators tested several top male-AGA loci in female cohorts—including regions on Xq12 (AR/EDA2R) and autosomal loci like 20p11, 7p21.1, 2q35, among others—most showed no significant association with FPHL (Redler et al. 2017). These results imply that while some genetic factors are shared, FPHL likely has distinct genetic determinants beyond those driving male baldness.Indeed, research indicates FPHL cannot be fully explained by androgen-mediated mechanisms alone. Non-androgenic pathways are thought to contribute. For example, signaling pathways like Wnt/β-catenin—crucial for hair follicle growth—may be modulated in pattern hair loss. Androgens are known to alter Wnt signaling in the scalp, potentially promoting miniaturization (Martinez-Jacobo et al. 2018). It has been hypothesized that dysregulation of Wnt signaling or other growth pathways could lead to follicle shrinkage even in the absence of high androgen levels. Additional evidence for androgen-independent factors comes from clinical observations: FPHL can occur in women without hyperandrogenism, and some women with FPHL do not respond to anti-androgen therapies (Fabbrocini et al. 2018). A study by Yip et al. (2009) also pointed to estrogen metabolism genes in FPHL—finding that a common variant in the aromatase gene (CYP19A1), associated with higher estrogen levels, was more frequent in women with FPHL

(Yip et al. 2009). This suggests that subtle differences in how androgens are converted to estrogens locally in the scalp might influence susceptibility to hair thinning (Yip et al. 2009).

Once the process is triggered, the histologic hallmark of both male and female-pattern loss is follicular miniaturization. Terminal (thick, long) hairs are gradually replaced by vellus-like (fine, short) hairs due to a shortened anagen phase and prolonged resting phase. In women, this miniaturization tends to be patchy and diffuse; complete bald areas are usually absent except in rare advanced cases (Fabbrocini et al. 2018). Scalp biopsies in FPHL classically show an increased proportion of thin vellus hairs and a decreased terminal:vellus hair ratio. (A normal scalp has a terminal:vellus ratio around 7:1, whereas an affected area in AGA may drop below 4:1 (Dhurat and Saraogi 2009). Often there is a mild perifollicular lymphocytic infiltration and fibrosis, sometimes termed '"microinflammation," around miniaturizing follicles (Dhurat and Saraogi 2009). This inflammatory component, while not scarring, suggests immune or microenvironmental factors contribute to follicle damage in pattern hair loss. Interestingly, one study noted that treatment with anti-androgens was more effective in FPHL patients whose ferritin (iron storage) levels were above 40 μg/L (Ramos and Miot 2015), highlighting how general health factors like iron deficiency or other micronutrient imbalances might modulate hair growth. Overall, the picture that emerges is that FPHL results from a combination of genetic sensitivity, hormonal effects (both androgenic and possibly estrogenic), and local follicular changes (microinflammation, altered signaling pathways) that together lead to progressive thinning. Moreover, hormonal dysregulation can accelerate this process. Women with conditions of androgen excess (e.g., PCOS, congenital adrenal hyperplasia) often experience earlier or more severe pattern hair loss due to increased DHT activity at the follicle (Carmina et al. 2019). Even without overt endocrine disorders, the natural hormonal shifts of aging have an effect: as described below, menopause brings a decline in estrogen and relative increase in androgenic influence, which can exacerbate follicle miniaturization. Conversely, the high estrogen milieu of pregnancy temporarily reverses miniaturization by prolonging the growth phase. These observations reinforce that while FPHL is not strictly "androgen-dependent" in the way male balding is, hormones still profoundly influence its course.

Epidemiology of FPHL

FPHL is the most common cause of hair loss in women, and its prevalence increases with age . However, reported prevalence ranges vary widely (6–38% in surveys of healthy women) due to differences in diagnostic criteria and populations studied (Fabbrocini et al. 2018). It is generally agreed that detectable FPHL is uncommon in women under 30, then rises steadily in later decades. One long-term study in the U.K. found that approximately 12% of women show signs of FPHL by age 29, 25% by age 49, and around 41% by age 69 (Birch et al. 2002). By age 79, more than half of women have some degree of hair thinning (Birch et al. 2002). In very advanced age, female-pattern loss becomes almost normative—only about 43% of women over 80 had no evidence of FPHL in one report (Sinclair and Dawber 2001). Interestingly, FPHL typically begins later in life than male-pattern hair loss. Whereas men often start balding in their 20s, women more commonly develop noticeable thinning in their 30s or 40s (i.e. during the reproductive years or peri-menopause) (Fabbrocini et al. 2018). Cases of severe teenage female-pattern alopecia are rare. When hair loss does present in younger women, it is often mild; other diagnoses like telogen effluvium or alopecia areata should be carefully ruled out in these patients (see "Prepubescent Period" below). That said, the psychological impact of even mild hair thinning can be significant for women in early adulthood. In fact, the demand for treatment is highest among women 25 to 40 years old, according to dermatology clinic data (Tosti and Piraccini, 2006). Many women seek medical advice as soon as they notice increased shedding or a wider part, reflecting the high cosmetic and emotional importance of hair for women in this age range. Ethnicity may also play a role in prevalence and presentation. Some studies (e.g., Ramos and Miot 2015) have noted variations among different ethnic groups, though universally age remains a key factor (Fabbrocini et al. 2018). Regardless of background, FPHL is a progressive condition. Without intervention, what begins as slight widening of the central part or reduced volume can advance to more diffuse thinning across the crown over years or decades. Fortunately, complete baldness is exceedingly uncommon in women—patients usually maintain at least a thin covering of hair even in advanced cases, which is a major difference from male baldness patterns.

Hormonal Influence on Female Hair Loss Across Different Life Stages

See Table 3.1.

Hormonal fluctuations throughout a woman's life have profound effects on the hair growth cycle. Below, we outline how hair characteristics and patterns of loss can change during various life stages, from birth through menopause (summarized from sources including Grymowicz et al. 2020 and others). Understanding these shifts is important for distinguishing normal physiologic changes from pathological hair loss, and for tailoring management of FPHL according to a patient's age and hormonal status.

Birth and Infancy

Newborn infants often enter the world with a full head of fine hair, only to lose much of it within the first few months of life. This phenomenon is a result of dramatic hormonal changes at birth.

Table 3.1 Influence of Hormones on the Hair Cycle in Different Stages of Female Life

Stage of Life	*Main Hormones Involved*	*Effect*
Puberty	Androgens	Transformation of vellus hair into terminal hair in the pubic and axillary regions
Reproductive age	Androgen excess (e.g., PCOS, NCAH, Cushing's syndrome, hyperprolactinemia)	Hirsutism
	Unknown/unexplained role of sex hormones	Female-pattern hair loss
	Hyperthyreosis	Alopecia areata
	Hypothyreosis	Diffuse alopecia
Pregnancy	High levels of estrogen, progesterone, prolactin, and growth factors	Increases in hair growth, hair diameter, and anagen/telogen
Puerperium	Decrease in estrogen and progesterone	Postpartum telogen effluvium
Menopause	Estrogen depletion	Female-pattern hair loss
		Facial hirsutism

Source: Adapted from Grymowicz et al. (2020).

In utero, the fetus is exposed to high levels of maternal hormones including estrogen (estradiol, estrone, and estriol) that cross the placenta and can promote hair follicles to stay in the growth phase. At birth, those maternal hormone levels drop rapidly. The sudden withdrawal triggers many of the infant's hair follicles to synchronously shift from anagen (growth) into telogen (resting), leading to increased shedding known as telogen effluvium of the newborn (Sarkar et al. 2024). Parents often notice their baby's hair thinning or bald patches developing around 2–3 months of age, which can be alarming but is a normal process. This "reset" of the hair cycle makes way for new hair growth as the infant's own endocrine system takes over regulation. Typically, hair lost in the neonatal period regrows by 6 to 12 months of age as hormone levels stabilize and follicles resume asynchronous cycling (Seattle Children's 2025). It's not unusual for the replacement hair to differ in texture or color from the newborn hair. Overall, unless other signs of illness are present, diffuse hair shedding in a 2- to 4-month-old baby is considered a benign, self-resolving condition caused by the drop in circulating estrogens after birth (Xu et al. 2017).

Prepubescent Period

In childhood (before puberty), pattern hair loss is exceedingly rare. Healthy prepubertal girls have abundant, thick scalp hair, and any significant hair thinning in this age group should prompt evaluation for other causes. When diffuse hair loss does occur in a young girl, it can present a diagnostic challenge—not only to worried parents, but also to physicians. Androgenetic alopecia is very uncommon prior to puberty (since significant androgen production has not yet begun); therefore, more likely explanations must be considered. Common causes of pediatric alopecia include tinea capitis (fungal infection), alopecia areata (autoimmune hair loss), telogen effluvium (often from illness or stress), and traction hair loss from pulling or styling (Figure 3.1) (Xu et al. 2017).

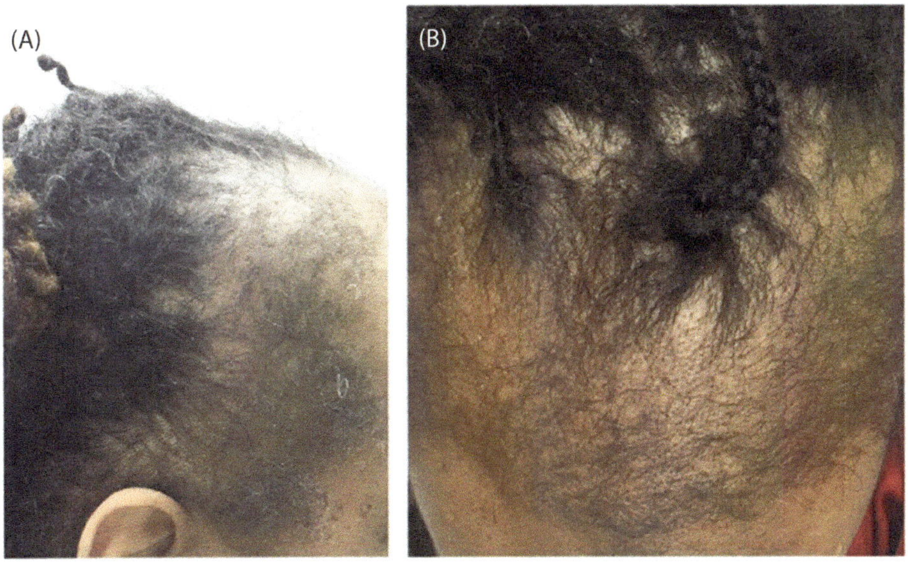

Figure 3.1 Clinical clues to traction alopecia in children/adolescents. (A) The "fringe sign"— a rim of retained fine hairs along the frontal hairline despite recession behind it. (B) "Tenting" of hair from tight braids/pigtails, with hairs pulled upward from the scalp. These patterns help distinguish traction alopecia from diffuse thinning disorders such as telogen effluvium or early androgenetic alopecia. Adapted from Xu L, Liu KX, Senna MM, 2017.

These can sometimes mimic the appearance of diffuse thinning. For example, acute telogen effluvium can cause a child's hair volume to decrease noticeably, and alopecia areata can rarely present as diffuse shedding instead of distinct patches. Distinguishing early AGA from these mimics is difficult based on visual exam alone in a child. Certain clues can aid in diagnosis. A family history of early-onset pattern baldness (in close male or female relatives) might raise suspicion for true androgenetic alopecia if a child shows gradual thinning. The progression of hair loss over time is also telling—AGA will slowly worsen, whereas telogen effluvium usually self-corrects once the trigger is resolved. Modern tools like dermoscopy (scalp microscopy) are valuable for evaluating pediatric hair loss. Dermoscopic findings such as variability in hair shaft diameter (greater than 20% diversity) and the presence of many miniaturized vellus hairs in the frontal scalp are supportive of AGA (Fabbrocini et al. 2018). These features would be absent in telogen effluvium, which instead shows uniformly short regrowing hairs and no miniaturization. In ambiguous cases, a scalp biopsy can be performed for definitive diagnosis. Histology of androgenetic alopecia in a child would show the characteristic increase in vellus hairs and miniaturized follicles. However, due to the invasive nature, biopsy is reserved for atypical cases or when an underlying disease is suspected and needs confirmation. In practice, if a prepubescent girl has slowly progressive diffuse thinning and other causes are ruled out, a diagnosis of "prepubertal pattern hair loss" might be made. Management is challenging given the young age, and often observation or minimal treatment is recommended until puberty, when the condition may accelerate and more standard therapies (like topical minoxidil) can be considered.

Puberty

Puberty brings a surge of adrenal and gonadal androgens, which has noticeable effects on hair throughout the body. In both sexes, rising androgens during adolescence transform vellus hair into terminal hair in certain areas – for example, in males androgens induce beard growth, and in all adolescents, pubic and axillary hair appears (conversion of vellus to terminal hair) under androgen influence (Grymowicz et al. 2020). However, in individuals with a genetic predisposition to androgenetic alopecia, these same hormones can trigger early manifestations of scalp hair thinning. It is uncommon but not unheard of for FPHL to begin in the teenage years. A girl genetically prone to pattern hair loss might notice a slight widening of the part or reduced volume in her late teens as androgen levels peak. Often this is initially mistaken for hairstyling issues or telogen effluvium from exam stress, etc. Over time, if the loss progresses, the pattern (diffuse central thinning with preserved frontal fringe) may become evident, confirming AGA. During puberty, clinicians must differentiate between true AGA and other common causes of diffuse hair loss in adolescents. As in younger children, telogen effluvium (TE) is a frequent culprit of shedding in this age group—for example, after crash dieting, a severe illness, or even the hormonal turbulence of puberty itself. Diffuse alopecia areata can also occur in teens, masquerading as pattern thinning (though careful exam might show subtle patchiness or exclamation-point hairs in alopecia areata). Usually, the progression of hair loss and presence of other signs of hyperandrogenism help make the diagnosis. In girls, signs like hirsutism, severe acne, irregular menses, or polycystic ovary syndrome (PCOS) may accompany early AGA, since excess androgens can contribute to all these conditions. PCOS in an adolescent female can present with both hirsutism (excess body hair) and pattern scalp hair loss – essentially a female analogue of male balding due to elevated androgen levels (Prasad et al. 2021). A careful history and hormonal work-up may be warranted if such signs are present.When female AGA is suspected in an adolescent, dermatologic evaluation is similar to

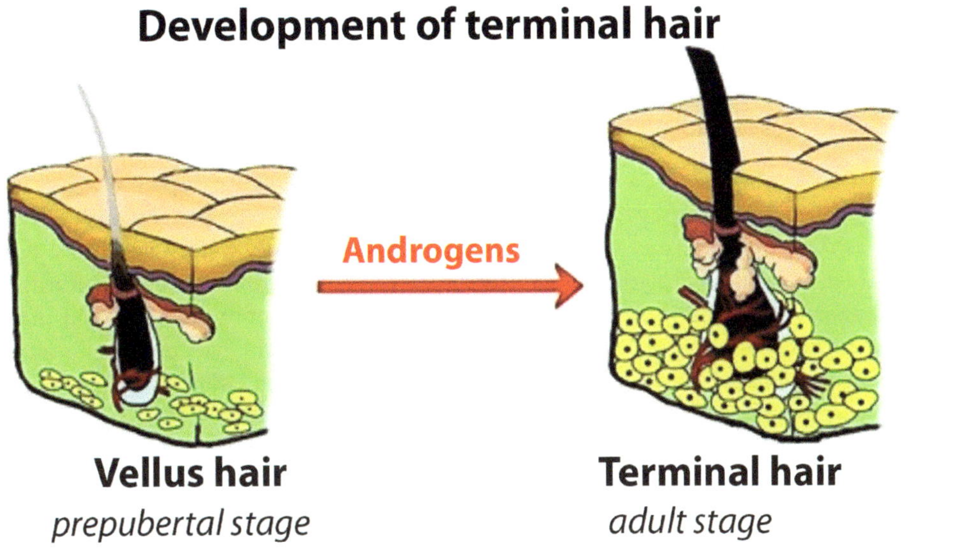

Figure 3.2 Development of terminal hair (from Kubek15/Wikipedia, under Creative Commons Attribution license).

adults. Dermoscopy can reveal hair shaft diameter variation and vellus hair increase on the crown, supportive of FPHL (Fabbrocini et al. 2018). A hair pull test might be mildly positive if active shedding is occurring, but not as strongly as in telogen effluvium (Fabbrocini et al. 2018). In most cases, an invasive biopsy can be avoided in teenagers; clinical monitoring over a few months will demonstrate whether miniaturization is progressing (confirming AGA) or whether the hair loss was transient. If a scalp biopsy is performed, diagnostic findings for AGA include a terminal:vellus hair ratio below 4:1 (normal is about 7:1) along with perifollicular fibrosis or inflammation around miniaturized follicles (Dhurat and Saraogi, 2009). Histologically, a ratio in the range of 3:1 or 4:1 strongly points to pattern hair loss rather than chronic telogen effluvium (Prasad et al. 2021). These changes reflect the androgen-driven shrinkage of follicles. Management of confirmed adolescent FPHL must be cautious—often focusing on topical minoxidil and treating any underlying endocrine disorder (like PCOS)—because many standard systemic treatments (e.g. oral finasteride or spironolactone) are not typically used until after puberty.

Pregnancy and Postpartum

Pregnancy is often described as a period of luxuriant hair growth for many women. This is because during pregnancy, high levels of estrogen, progesterone, prolactin, and placental growth factors create a hormonal environment that favors hair retention. Estrogen in particular prolongs the anagen phase of the hair cycle, meaning fewer hairs transition to shedding mode. Women in late pregnancy have been shown to have an increased anagen-to-telogen ratio—more hairs than usual are in the active growth phase (Grover and Khurana, 2013). Clinically, this translates to thicker, fuller hair. Many expectant mothers notice their hair feels denser and sheds very little during the second and third trimesters. The scalp follicles essentially synchronize in staying in anagen under the influence of pregnancy hormones (Grover and Khurana, 2013). Additionally, as mentioned earlier, estrogen enhances scalp circulation; the vasodilation improves nutrient delivery to follicles, further supporting robust growth (Rinaldi et al. 2023). This hormonal reprieve from shedding is temporary, however. Shortly after childbirth, the endocrine balance swings back: estrogen and progesterone levels plummet with the delivery of the placenta.

The result of this sudden hormonal withdrawal in the postpartum period is a well-known phenomenon called postpartum telogen effluvium (also termed telogen gravidarum). With the protective effect of estrogen gone, a large number of hairs that were artificially prolonged in anagen now enter telogen together. Approximately 3 to 4 months after delivery, women experience diffuse shedding as those synchronized telogen hairs are released from the scalp (Grover and Khurana, 2013). This can be quite dramatic—clumps of hair coming out in the shower or hairbrush—and understandably distressing to new mothers. The hair loss is most noticeable around the frontal scalp (sometimes producing a thin fringe or "baby hairs" along the hairline) but in fact affects the entire scalp globally. The good news is that postpartum telogen effluvium is temporary. Peak shedding occurs around 3–4 months postpartum and then gradually abates. In most cases, the hair density returns to its pre-pregnancy baseline by about 6 to 12 months after childbirth, once the normal hair cycle resumes (Mirmirani, 2011). Breastfeeding does not prevent this process (since it is driven by hormone changes after pregnancy), though some anecdotal reports suggest it might prolong the shedding phase slightly. Ultimately, postpartum hair loss represents the body "catching up" on the hairs that were retained during pregnancy. Dermatologists reassure patients that this is a self-limited process of regrowth following synchronized shedding, and treatment is usually not required other than cosmetic measures and nutritional support (to ensure factors like iron or thyroid are normal, as deficiencies can worsen the shedding).

Menopause

Menopause is a critical turning point for hair in many women. The hormonal milieu shifts significantly—primarily through a steep decline in estrogen levels—and this has direct repercussions on the hair follicle's health and cycling. Estrogen has multiple beneficial effects on hair: it prolongs the growth phase, supports the dermal papilla cells, and improves scalp vascularization as noted earlier (Rinaldi et al. 2023). When estrogen levels fall during menopause, these protective mechanisms wane. Follicles tend to have shorter anagen phases and longer telogen phases, meaning hairs grow more slowly and shed more readily. Clinically, many postmenopausal women notice a progressive diffuse thinning in the frontal and crown areas, even if they had relatively thick hair before. The hair shaft diameter may also reduce (individual hairs become finer). This menopausal thinning is essentially an acceleration of FPHL, and it often becomes more apparent in the decade after menopause. In fact, epidemiological data show a marked jump in FPHL prevalence in women over age 50, correlating with the menopausal transition (Gupta et al. 2025).

A key factor is the change in the balance between estrogens and androgens. Unlike estrogens, androgen production declines more gradually with age in women, and the ovaries continue to produce small amounts of testosterone even after menopause. The result is a higher androgen-to-estrogen ratio in postmenopausal women (Rinaldi et al. 2023). Even though absolute androgen levels are not very high, the relative lack of estrogen's counterbalancing effect allows androgens (like DHT) to exert greater influence on susceptible follicles (Rinaldi et al. 2023). This can lead to a presentation that mirrors male-pattern baldness in some women—for example, more pronounced thinning at the vertex or even slight bitemporal recession—although true bald spots are still rare in females (Fabbrocini et al. 2018). The increase in relative androgen activity contributes to what some researchers call "clinical hyperandrogenism" in menopausal women: signs can include sebaceous gland hypertrophy (oilier scalp/skin) and accelerated FPHL (Rinaldi et al.

2023). Essentially, the hormonal shift tilts the scalp's environment toward one that favors hair follicle miniaturization (and sebum production) similar to the effect in genetically prone men.

Beyond hormones, metabolic and age-related factors during menopause also impact hair. As women age, there is reduced mitochondrial efficiency and impaired energy metabolism in cells throughout the body, including the hair follicle. Hair follicles are highly energy-demanding, and research shows they require substantial metabolic input to continuously grow hair fibers (Rinaldi et al. 2023). In menopause, slower metabolism and potential nutritional deficiencies can leave follicles with less energy and building blocks for hair production. Additionally, aging and estrogen loss are associated with increased oxidative stress and microinflammation in tissues. In scalp hair follicles, scientists have observed low-grade lymphocytic inflammatory infiltrates around follicles in FPHL (the "microinflammation" mentioned earlier) (Fabbrocini et al. 2018). This type of chronic inflammation can further disrupt the normal hair cycle and contribute to fibrosis (scarring) around follicles over time. Menopause appears to exacerbate these processes—some authors have even proposed the concept of a "hair follicle menopause," wherein follicles themselves undergo changes independent of systemic menopause, due to local metabolic and receptor changes (Rinaldi et al. 2023). For instance, one study found postmenopausal women with FPHL had significantly lower estrogen and higher DHT levels within scalp skin compared to postmenopausal women without hair loss (Fabbrocini et al. 2018), suggesting a local hormonal imbalance in affected follicles.Comorbid conditions common in mid-life can compound the issue. Metabolic syndrome, insulin resistance, and PCOS (if the latter persists into perimenopause) all can elevate androgens or inflammatory cytokines that negatively affect hair (El Sayed et al. 2016). Thyroid disorders, particularly the hypothyroidism that is more prevalent with age, can cause diffuse hair loss or contribute to thinning if not corrected. Furthermore, nutrient deficiencies are not uncommon in menopausal women – iron deficiency may arise from chronic low-level blood loss or dietary factors, and vitamin D deficiency is widespread. Both iron and vitamin D are important for follicle function (for example, iron is required for cell proliferation, and vitamin D has receptors in hair follicles). Ensuring adequate ferritin (iron stores) and vitamin D levels may help support hair growth during menopause, and many clinicians will check these in women presenting with hair thinning (Ramos and Miot, 2015).

Figure 3.3 shows Frontal fibrosing alopecia in a postmenopausal woman—an example of a scarring alopecia that can accompany or be mistaken for FPHL. Panel (a) shows recession of the frontal hairline; (b) lateral view of temporal loss; (c) loss of eyebrows. Panel (d) is a scalp biopsy image with perifollicular lymphocytic infiltrates and fibrosis around hair follicles (histological features characteristic of FFA). FFA primarily affects women after menopause and is considered a lichen planopilaris variant.

Female-pattern hair loss is a complex, multifaceted condition influenced by genetic, hormonal, and environmental factors that vary across a woman's life. Unlike male-pattern baldness, which is largely androgen-driven, FPHL involves a more diffuse thinning with generally preserved hairline and can occur even in the absence of overt androgen excess. This necessitates a tailored approach to diagnosis and treatment. A thorough history (including hormonal symptoms and life events), clinical examination with tools like dermoscopy, and selective laboratory tests form the cornerstone of evaluation to exclude other causes. Treatment often requires a combination of therapies addressing different pathogenic factors—for example, topical minoxidil to stimulate follicles, anti-androgens (systemic or topical) to counter DHT in patients with signs of hyperandrogenism, and nutritional or lifestyle modifications to optimize hair growth conditions. Psychosocial support is also crucial, as hair loss in women can significantly impact self-esteem and quality of life. Encouragingly, advances in research are continuously shedding light on the molecular and

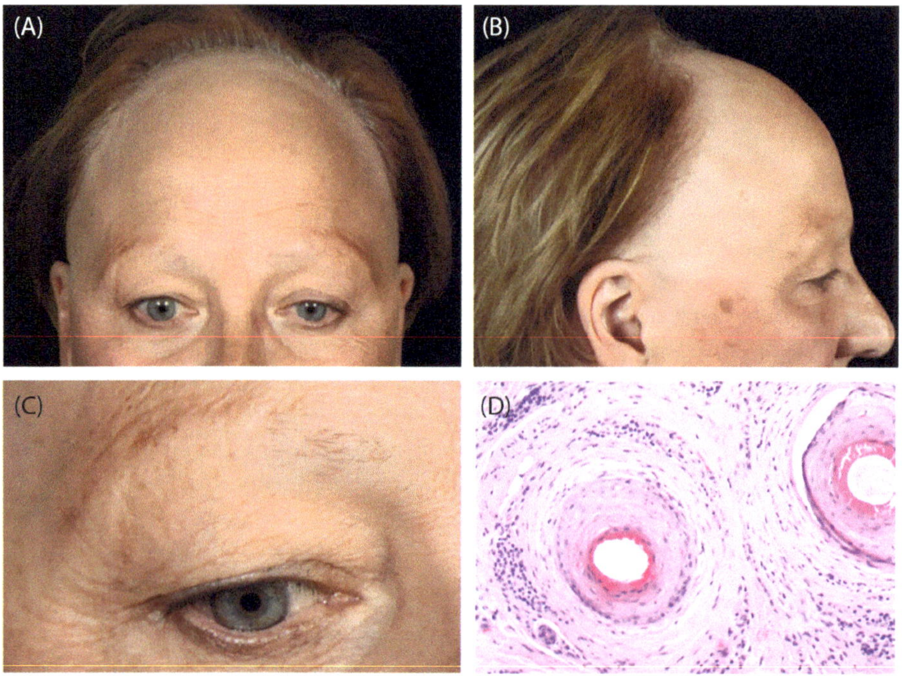

Figure 3.3 Fibrosing alopecia. (From C Tziotzios et al., Genome-wide association study in frontal fibrosing alopecia identifies four susceptibility loci including HLA-B*07:02, *Nat Commun* 2019;10:1150, under Creative Commons Attribution license.)

genetic underpinnings of FPHL. As we better understand the roles of specific genes, local growth factors, and immune components in female hair loss, new targeted therapies are likely to emerge from Wnt pathway modulators to agents that mimic estrogen's follicle-protective effects without systemic side effects.

In summary, FPHL is not simply "male balding in women"—it is a distinct entity that demands gender-specific considerations. By accounting for hormonal milestones (such as puberty, pregnancy, and menopause) and the unique pattern of female hair thinning, clinicians can provide personalized, effective care. With the rising interest in non-surgical treatments among women, ongoing research and patient education remain paramount. Understanding the biology of female hair loss across the lifespan will enable healthcare providers to not only improve hair density, but also restore confidence and quality of life for millions of affected women around the world.

Chapter 4

Clinical Scales for Hair Loss

Bilal F. Hamzeh, Haley Guinan, Julyssa A. Renteria and Robert Dorfman

Introduction

With the inherent complexity of hair loss diagnosis and treatment, the utilization of standardized scales to assess the extent and pattern of hair loss is crucial. Among these, the Norwood, Ludwig, and Savin scales are key elements in the initial diagnosis of hair loss in addition to assessing changes resulting from treatment.

The Norwood Scale, developed in the 1970s, categorizes male-pattern baldness into seven stages, ranging from minimal hair loss to advanced balding. It has become the gold standard in assessing androgenetic alopecia in men. Conversely, the Ludwig and Savin scales address female-pattern hair loss, which often presents more diffusely than in male patients, focusing on the degree of hair thinning on the crown and top of the head.

The Norwood–Hamilton Scale

The first standardized system for grading male-pattern hair loss (MPHL) was the Hamilton Scale, which was developed through observations of over 300 Male patients. The major categorizations of the Hamilton Scale are types I–III, which are less severe, and types IV–VII, which are more severe or effectively bald. The Hamilton Scale did have limitations: type III MPHL was described as borderline cases that were difficult to categorize into other stages, meaning the Hamilton Scale could not effectively grade every case of MPHL (Wirya et al. 2017). Moreover, the Hamilton Scale was developed based on observations of mostly Caucasian males, limiting application to other races and ethnicities (Gupta and Mysore 2016).

Building from the Hamilton Scale, the Norwood–Hamilton Scale was developed to further refine and categorize MPHL into discrete stages (Figure 4.1). After being developed in 1975, the Norwood–Hamilton Scale has continued to be the most widely used clinical scale for MPHL.

The Norwood–Hamilton Scale is thus a standardized system to grade the extent of androgenetic alopecia clinically, informing treatment approaches and assessing outcomes. The Norwood–Hamilton Scale consists of seven primary stages, each representing a different level of hair loss

DOI: 10.1201/9781032726397-4

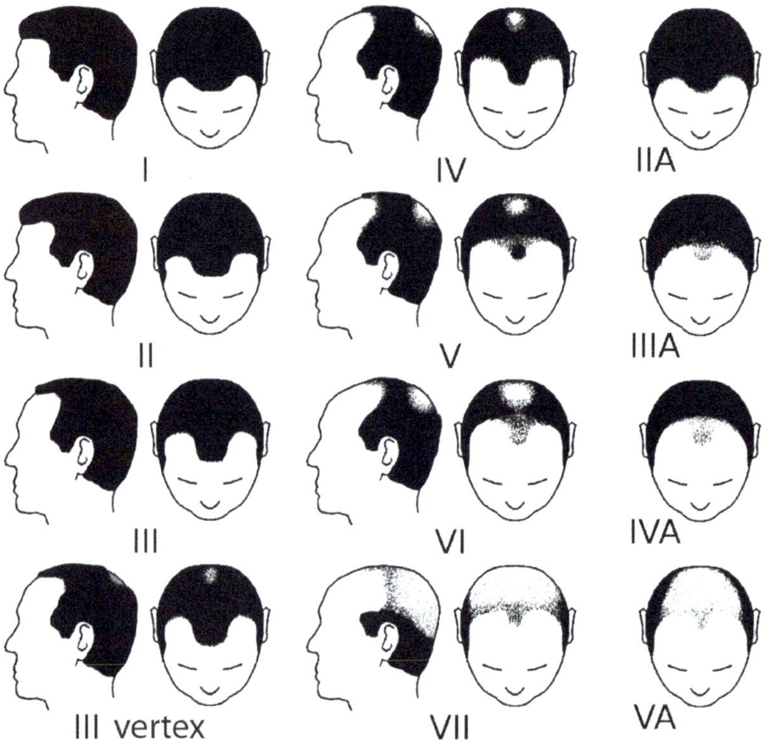

Figure 4.1 Norwood–Hamilton Scale (from Keminski/Wikipedia under Creative Commons license).

severity. Understanding these stages is crucial for both clinicians and patients, as they guide treatment decisions and help set realistic expectations.

- Stage I: Minimal or No Hair Loss
  - At this stage, there is little to no noticeable hair loss. The hairline remains largely intact, with only slight thinning, if any, along the temples.
- Stage II: Early Recession
  - Hair loss begins to manifest with a mild recession of the hairline around the temples, creating an M-shaped pattern. This stage is often considered the earliest visible sign of androgenetic alopecia.
- Stage III: Deeper Recession and Thinning
  - Hair loss becomes more pronounced, with deeper recession at the temples and thinning at the crown. Stage III is typically when patients first seek clinical advice, as the changes become more noticeable.
- Stage IV: Extensive Hair Loss at the Crown
  - The hairline continues to recede, and a distinct bald spot begins to form at the crown. The two areas of hair loss—temple recession and crown thinning—are usually still separated by a band of hair across the top of the head.
- Stage V: Bridging of Hair Loss Areas
  - As hair loss progresses, the band of hair separating the receding hairline and the crown thinning begins to narrow. The two areas may start to merge, creating a larger bald area.

- Stage VI: Advanced Baldness
  - The bridge of hair connecting the crown and the front hairline is now lost, leading to a more significant and continuous bald area. The remaining hair on the sides of the head may also begin to thin.
- Stage VII: Severe Baldness
  - The most severe form of male-pattern baldness, stage 7, is characterized by extensive hair loss across the top of the head. Only a narrow band of hair remains around the sides and back of the head.

The Norwood Scale helps clinicians identify the extent of hair loss and differentiate androgenetic alopecia (AGA) from other forms of alopecia, such as alopecia areata or telogen effluvium, which do not adhere to the same patterned hair loss as is observed in AGA. Although hair loss exhibits significant interpatient variability, the Norwood-Hamilton Scale is a vital tool in the clinical assessment, monitoring, and treatment of AGA.

The Ludwig Scale

Female-pattern hair loss (FPHL) presents differently from male-pattern baldness and requires distinct diagnostic criteria. The Ludwig Scale is the most widely used tool for assessing and categorizing hair loss in women, which primarily presents as diffuse thinning of hair across the scalp, particularly at the crown. Developed specifically to address the unique patterns of hair thinning observed in female patients, the Ludwig Scale provides clinicians with a standardized method for diagnosing the severity of hair loss and guiding treatment decisions. The Ludwig Scale is divided into three primary stages, each representing a different degree of hair thinning. This scale emphasizes the diffuse nature of female-pattern hair loss, where hair thinning occurs more uniformly across the scalp rather than in specific localized areas (Figure 4.2).

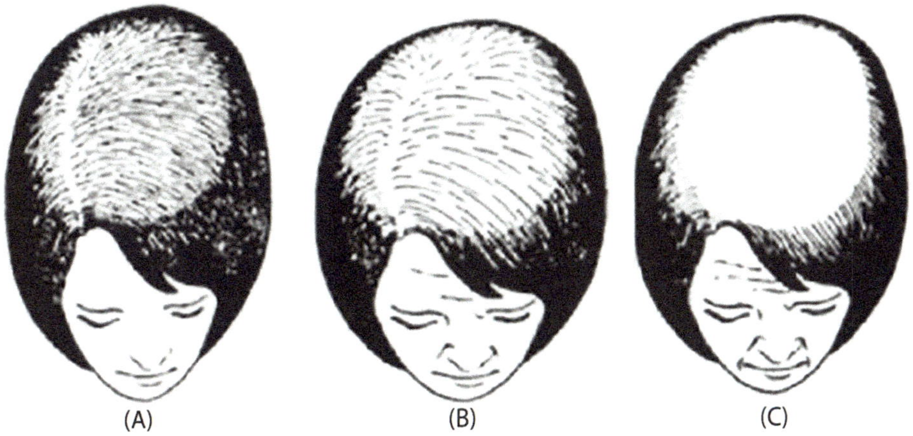

Figure 4.2 Ludwig Scale representation of female-pattern hair loss, illustrating the three grades of hair thinning. (A) Grade I: Perceptible thinning at the crown, limited by a line 1–3 cm behind the frontal hairline. (B) Grade II: Pronounced thinning on the crown within the area seen in Grade I. (C) Grade III: Full baldness covering the areas seen in grades I and II. (From G Fabbrocini et al., Female pattern hair loss: A clinical, pathophysiologic, and therapeutic review, *Int J Womens Dermatol*, 2018;4(4):203–211, with permission).

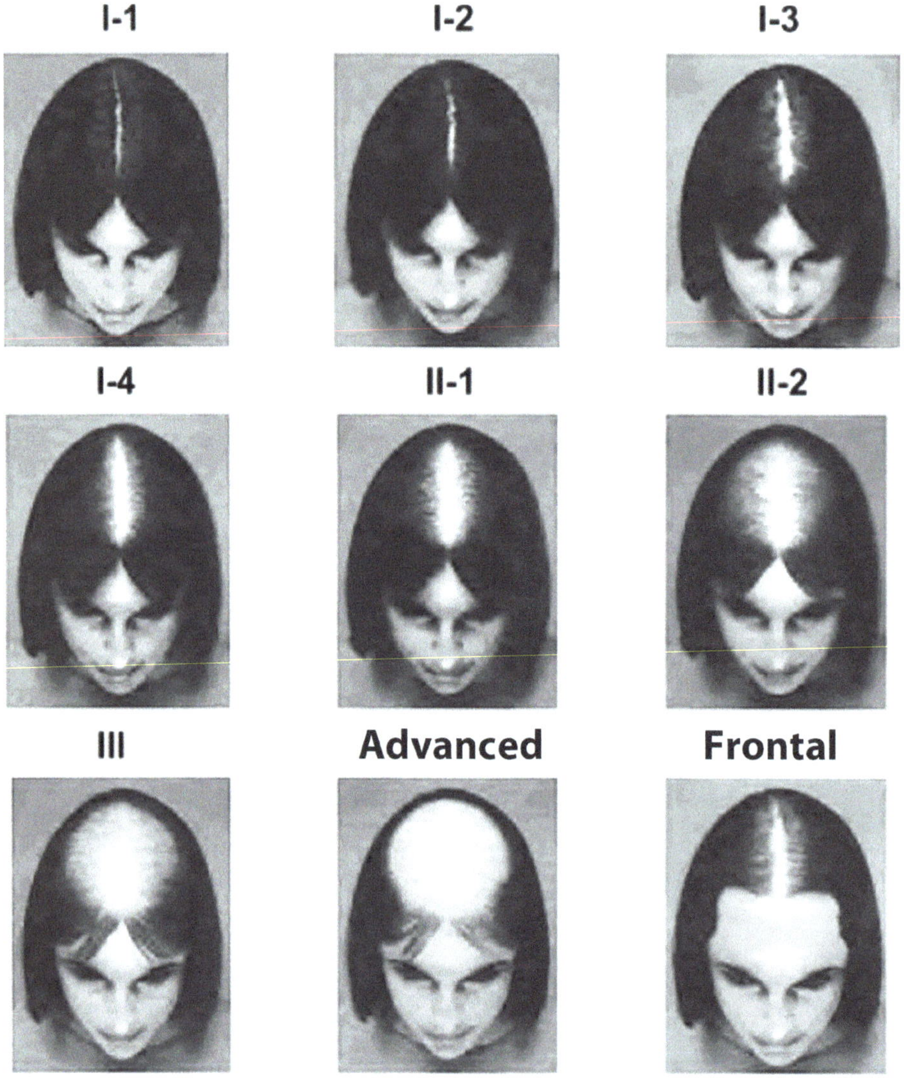

Figure 4.3 Savin Scale depicting a more detailed progression of FPHL relative to the Ludwig Scale, accounting for diffuse thinning along the part line and crown. Stage I shows slight thinning at the crown and along the part line with minimal visible scalp. Stage II exhibits more noticeable thinning, particularly along the part line. Progression through stage III shows pronounced crown thinning, aligning with Ludwig grade II. Advanced stages show significant hair loss at the crown and apex with retention of the frontal hairline, aligning with Ludwig grade III. (From RC Savin, *Evaluating androgenetic alopecia in male and female patients*, Kalamazoo, MI: The Upjohn Company, 1994).

1. Stage I: Mild Thinning
   - In the early stage of FPHL, hair thinning is generally mild and often goes unnoticed. The central parting of the hair may become slightly wider, and there may be a reduction in hair volume. However, the frontal hairline remains largely unaffected, and the overall appearance of the scalp is still relatively full.

2. Stage II: Moderate Thinning
   - At this stage, hair thinning becomes more noticeable, especially at the crown. The central part of the scalp shows significant thinning, and the widening of the central part line becomes more apparent. While the frontal hairline remains mostly intact, the overall density of the hair is reduced, leading to a more visible scalp.
3. Stage III: Severe Thinning
   - In the most advanced stage of the Ludwig Scale, the thinning at the crown becomes severe, and the scalp is prominently visible through the hair. The hair density across the top of the scalp is significantly diminished, and the widening of the central part is extensive. However, even in this stage, the frontal hairline is usually preserved, distinguishing FPHL from male-pattern baldness.

While the Ludwig Scale is a valuable tool, it does have limitations. The scale primarily focuses on the extent of visible thinning and does not account for other important factors such as hair density, texture, or variability in female alopecia patterns, which may not all follow the central parting observed in most patients. The Savin Scale is also utilized, staging similar hair loss patterns in female patients, but accounts for thinning and density in addition to patterning (Figure 4.3).

Scaling systems including but not limited to the Norwood-Hamilton, Ludwig, and Savin scales exhibit limitations pertaining to interpatient variability in presentation and alignment with diverse etiologies but continue to play a vital role in the diagnosis and monitoring of hair loss by both patients and practitioners.

Chapter 5

Other Pharmacotherapies

Haley Guinan, Julyssa A. Renteria and Robert Dorfman

Introduction

Hormonal treatments play a key role in the management of hair loss, particularly in cases where androgen sensitivity or hormonal imbalances are contributing factors. These therapies target the hormonal pathways that drive hair thinning, aiming to stabilize or reverse the progression of hair loss while promoting the growth of healthy, resilient hair. This chapter delves into the intricate relationship between hormones and hair health, highlighting the roles of key hormones and their mechanisms of action. It offers an in-depth examination of available hormonal therapies, including systemic and topical options, and their application in clinical practice. Case studies and clinical outcomes are presented to illustrate the practical benefits and limitations of these treatments.

Role of Hormones in Hair Loss

The intricate interplay between various hormones, particularly androgens, estrogens, thyroid hormones, cortisol, and insulin-like growth factor-1 (IGF-1), profoundly impacts the hair growth cycle and follicular health. A clear understanding of these hormonal mechanisms is essential for devising effective therapeutic strategies for hair loss.

Androgens

Androgens, such as testosterone and its more potent metabolite, dihydrotestosterone (DHT), are the primary hormones implicated in the development of androgenetic alopecia, also known as male or female-pattern hair loss. Androgens exert their effects on the hair follicles through the androgen receptor (AR), which is expressed in the dermal papilla cells and outer root sheath cells of the follicle (Kaufman 2002). In genetically susceptible individuals, the binding of DHT to the AR triggers a cascade of events that leads to follicular miniaturization, shortening of the anagen (growth) phase, and progressive hair thinning.

 DOI: 10.1201/9781032726397-5

Estrogens

Estrogens, such as estradiol and estrone, are female sex hormones that have a protective effect on hair growth. They counteract androgen activity by prolonging the anagen phase (Ohnemus et al. 2006) and modulating androgen metabolism via aromatase, which converts androgens to estrogens. Estrogens, particularly 17β-estradiol (E2), exert their effects on hair follicles by binding to the estrogen receptors (ERs) expressed within them. This interaction regulates gene activity and aids in metabolizing androgens in the pilosebaceous unit (Ohnemus et al. 2006). Moreover, estrogens boost aromatase enzyme activity, which converts androgens into estrogens, thereby lowering DHT levels—a key contributor to androgenetic alopecia (AGA) (Hoffman et al. 2002). They are also known to influence the phases of the hair cycle. During pregnancy, higher estrogen levels result in prolonged growth phases and thicker hair, while the postpartum estrogen decline is associated with temporary hair shedding (Wallace 1998). Preclinical studies reinforce this role, showing that ovariectomized (OVX) mice, which lack endogenous estrogen, experience hair regrowth and increased density when supplemented with E2 (Endo et al. 2018). The decline in estrogen levels during menopause can contribute to hair thinning in women, as the balance between estrogens and androgens shifts in favor of the latter.

Thyroid Hormones

Thyroid hormones, including thyroxine (T4) and triiodothyronine (T3), play a vital role in regulating hair growth and maintaining hair follicle health. Imbalances in thyroid function, such as hypothyroidism or hyperthyroidism, can lead to hair loss, often presenting as diffuse thinning or telogen effluvium (Paus and Cotsarelis 1999). These conditions typically improve with appropriate medical treatment to normalize thyroid levels. Mechanistically, T3 and T4 directly stimulate hair matrix keratinocyte proliferation and prolong the anagen (growth) phase by suppressing anagen-inhibitory factors like TGF-beta 2 and modulating thyroid-responsive keratins, such as CK6 and CK14 (van Beek 2008). They also regulate stem cell activity within hair follicles by promoting keratin 15 expression and enhancing CD200, an immune-inhibitory molecule, which may protect against autoimmune-mediated hair loss like alopecia areata (AA) (Tiede 2010). Additionally, T3 and T4 improve mitochondrial function and reduce oxidative stress in hair follicles, supporting their energy needs and overall health, which is essential for sustaining robust hair growth and quality (Vidali 2014).

Cortisol

Cortisol, a glucocorticoid hormone produced by the adrenal glands, is integral to the body's stress response. Elevated cortisol levels, often resulting from chronic stress, have been linked to hair loss, particularly telogen effluvium (Arck et al. 2003), where hair follicles prematurely transition from the anagen (growth) phase to the telogen (resting) phase, leading to increased hair shedding. Cortisol disrupts hair follicle function by reducing the synthesis and accelerating the breakdown of essential skin components like hyaluronan and proteoglycans, compromising follicle health (Thom 2016). It also adversely affects dermal papilla cells (DPCs), decreasing their proliferation and expression of growth factors such as Wnt5a, alkaline phosphatase (ALP), and vascular endothelial growth factor (VEGF), contributing to follicular miniaturization and hair loss (Lee

2017). Moreover, cortisol and synthetic glucocorticoids, such as dexamethasone, can enhance AR activity in DPCs, exacerbating AGA by intensifying the suppressive effects of androgens on hair growth (Kwack et al. 2022). The hypothalamic–pituitary–adrenal (HPA) axis also plays a critical role in stress-induced hair loss, particularly in autoimmune conditions like AA (Ito 2005). Stress activates the HPA axis, elevating corticotropin-releasing hormone (CRH) and adrenocorticotropic hormone (ACTH), which increase cortisol production. This dysregulation contributes to autoimmune-mediated follicular damage, further accelerating hair loss in AA.

Insulin and Insulin-Like Growth Factor-1 (IGF-1)

Insulin and insulin-like growth factor-1 (IGF-1) play pivotal roles in the regulation of hair growth and the maintenance of hair follicle health. Insulin resistance and hyperinsulinemia, commonly associated with conditions such as polycystic ovary syndrome (PCOS) and metabolic syndrome, can contribute to hair loss in both men and women (Matilainen et al. 2001). IGF-1, a growth factor structurally similar to insulin, has been shown to stimulate hair follicle proliferation and prolong the anagen phase, making it integral to healthy hair growth. In AGA, IGF-1 is essential for the proliferation and differentiation of DPCs. The AR pathway, however, can suppress IGF-1 expression through the promotion of miR-221 transcription (Li et al. 2023; He et al. 2022). This suppression inactivates the MAPK and PI3K/AKT pathways in DPCs and dermal sheath cells, leading to reduced hair growth and follicle miniaturization. Additionally, overexpression of miR-122 in AGA directly induces apoptosis of DPCs by targeting the IGF-1 receptor, further exacerbating hair loss. Although the role of IGF-1 in AA is less documented than in AGA, it is known to support hair follicle health by promoting the anagen phase and inhibiting apoptosis. The autoimmune destruction of hair follicles seen in AA may indirectly impact IGF-1's ability to support follicle survival and growth due to the inflammatory environment. Overall, IGF-1 signaling is crucial for maintaining the hair growth cycle and follicular differentiation. It facilitates the transition from the telogen (resting) phase to the anagen (growth) phase and supports the structural integrity of hair follicles (Weger and Schlake 2005). Reduced IGF-1 levels in DPCs from balding scalp follicles have been associated with male-pattern baldness, emphasizing its role in hair follicle biology (Panchaprateep and Asawanonda 2014).

The hormonal regulation of hair growth reflects a complex and interconnected system. Addressing hormonal imbalances and modulating their effects on hair follicles is crucial for developing targeted treatments. A comprehensive understanding of these pathways (Table 5.1) allows practitioners to design tailored therapies, effectively managing hair loss and supporting the growth of healthy, resilient hair.

Hormonal Therapies for Hair Restoration

Hormonal therapies for hair restoration aim to address the underlying hormonal factors contributing to hair loss, particularly in cases of androgenetic alopecia and other hormone-related hair disorders. These therapies can be broadly categorized into systemic treatments, which target hormonal imbalances throughout the body, and topical treatments, which act directly on the hair follicles.

Table 5.1 Hormonal Effects on Hair Growth

Hormone	*Effect on Hair Growth*	*Mechanism of Action*	*Associated Conditions*
Androgens (e.g., testosterone, DHT)	Contribute to follicular miniaturization, hair thinning, and androgenetic alopecia	Bind to androgen receptors in hair follicles, triggering follicular miniaturization and shortened anagen phase	Androgenetic alopecia (male/female-pattern hair loss)
Estrogens (e.g., estradiol)	Protective effect; prolong anagen phase	Counteract androgen action and enhance follicle health	Hair thinning during menopause due to decreased estrogen levels
Thyroid hormones (T3, T4)	Maintain follicle health; imbalance can cause diffuse thinning or telogen effluvium	Regulate hair growth and metabolic activity in follicles	Hypothyroidism, hyperthyroidism
Cortisol	Stress-induced hair loss (telogen effluvium)	Induces premature transition of follicles from anagen to telogen phase	Chronic stress
Insulin and IGF-1	Stimulate hair follicle proliferation; insulin resistance can impair hair health	Promote anagen phase via metabolic and growth factor pathways	PCOS, metabolic syndrome, insulin resistance

Systemic Treatments

5-Alpha Reductase Inhibitors

5-Alpha reductase inhibitors, including finasteride and dutasteride, are cornerstone treatments for AGA in men, targeting the hormonal pathways that drive hair follicle miniaturization. These medications function by inhibiting the conversion of testosterone to dihydrotestosterone (DHT), a potent androgen implicated in the pathogenesis of AGA (Kaufman et al. 1998). By reducing DHT levels, these inhibitors slow hair loss and promote the regrowth of terminal hair. These inhibitors specifically target the type II isoenzyme of 5-alpha reductase, which converts testosterone to DHT (Dhurat et al. 2020). DHT binds to androgen receptors in dermal papilla cells, initiating processes that result in hair follicle miniaturization. By blocking this conversion, finasteride and dutasteride effectively decrease scalp and serum DHT levels, mitigating androgen-mediated damage and supporting the restoration of hair follicle health. Finasteride, at a dosage of 1 mg daily (U.S. National Library of Medicine 2024), has been extensively studied and shown to significantly improve hair density, thickness, and count in men with AGA). Dutasteride, which inhibits both type I and type II isoenzymes, has demonstrated superior efficacy in reducing DHT levels and promoting hair regrowth compared to finasteride (Olsen et al. 2006). Clinical trials demonstrate sustained efficacy over 12 months or more with continued use. Finasteride is administered at 1 mg daily, with or without meals. Consistent use for at least 3 months is required to observe benefits, and continued treatment is essential to maintain results, as discontinuation often leads to reversal of effects within 12 months. Dutasteride, while not FDA approved for AGA in the US, is available in some countries and used off-label at dosages of 0.5 mg daily. Both finasteride and dutasteride have favorable safety profiles. The most common side effects are mild and include sexual dysfunction, such as decreased libido, erectile dysfunction, and ejaculation disorders, which are typically reversible upon discontinuation. Long-term studies have not demonstrated significant effects on hormone levels or the hypothalamic–pituitary–testicular axis, further supporting their safety for prolonged use in the management of AGA.

Antiandrogens

Antiandrogens, such as spironolactone and cyproterone acetate, are commonly used in the treatment of female-pattern hair loss (Starace et al. 2020). These medications work by blocking the action of androgens at the receptor level, thereby reducing the androgen-mediated damage to the hair follicles (Sinclair et al. 2005). Spironolactone, at dosages ranging from 50 to 200 mg per day, has been shown to be effective in reducing hair loss and promoting hair regrowth in women with androgenetic alopecia (Rathnayake and Sinclair 2010). Before initiating hormonal therapy, a thorough examination of the female patient is required, including a urine pregnancy test followed by a confirmatory serum beta-hCG test. It is also important to assess the patient's overall health, hormonal status, and suitability for hormonal therapy. Baseline blood tests, such as electrolyte levels and kidney function, should be conducted, as spironolactone and cyproterone acetate can impact potassium levels and renal function (Coneac et al. 2014). Recent studies have identified novel topical AR antagonists, such as compound 30a, which promote hair growth in both AGA mouse models and hair-growth models without notable systemic toxicity (H. Zhang et al. 2024). These findings suggest the potential of targeted topical therapies to address androgen activity in the scalp while minimizing systemic side effects. RU58841, a non-steroidal antiandrogen, has shown promising results in controlled studies (De Brouwer et al. 1997). Using balding scalp grafts maintained on testosterone-conditioned nude mice, RU58841-treated grafts demonstrated higher numbers of active follicles and enhanced linear hair growth rates compared to untreated controls, highlighting its efficacy in stimulating hair growth. Flutamide, tested in topical formulations, has shown significant improvements in hair density, length, and diameter in human bald scalp grafts transplanted onto SCID mice (Sintov et al. 2000). Comparative studies revealed that flutamide-treated grafts produced more hair per graft and longer hair shafts than those treated with finasteride or placebo.

Oral Contraceptives

Oral contraceptives, which combine estrogen and progestin, are often used to manage female-pattern hair loss, particularly in women with underlying hormonal conditions such as PCOS. The estrogen component counteracts androgen effects on hair follicles, while the progestin component reduces androgen production by the ovaries (Riedel-Baima and Riedel 2008). These mechanisms contribute to their effectiveness in treating AGA by lowering androgen levels and blocking androgen receptor activity. Combined oral contraceptives suppress the secretion of gonadotropin-releasing hormone (GnRH), follicle-stimulating hormone (FSH), and luteinizing hormone (LH). This suppression decreases ovarian androgen production and increases sex hormone-binding globulin (SHBG) levels. SHBG binds free testosterone, reducing its availability to activate androgen receptors. Certain progestins in oral contraceptives, such as norgestimate and dienogest, inhibit the enzyme 5-alpha reductase, which converts testosterone into DHT (Rabe et al. 2000). By decreasing DHT levels, these progestins help mitigate hair follicle miniaturization associated with AGA. Progestins such as cyproterone acetate and drospirenone possess antiandrogenic properties that directly block androgen receptors in hair follicles, thereby reducing androgen-induced hair loss (Williams et al. 2021). Clinical studies have shown that treatment with cyproterone acetate combined with ethinyl estradiol significantly improves hair density in women with diffuse androgen-dependent alopecia, particularly when ferritin levels are sufficient (Rushton and Ramsay 1992). Drospirenone, an analog of spironolactone, combined with ethinyl estradiol, has been effective in lowering androgen levels and enhancing hair density in women with AGA (Reynolds 2024). By modulating androgen activity, oral contraceptives offer a targeted approach to addressing hormone-related hair loss in women, with promising outcomes in clinical settings.

Topical Treatments

Topical Finasteride

Topical formulations of finasteride have emerged as a viable alternative to oral finasteride, aiming to reduce systemic side effects while retaining therapeutic efficacy. Research has shown that topical finasteride, at concentrations ranging from 0.005% to 0.1%, can enhance hair growth and decrease hair loss in men with AGA (Suchonwanit et al. 2019). Evidence from a phase III randomized controlled trial demonstrated that topical finasteride spray solution significantly increased target area hair count (TAHC) at 24 weeks (Piraccini et al. 2022). These results were comparable to those achieved with oral finasteride but with significantly reduced systemic absorption and a smaller impact on serum DHT levels. This indicates that topical finasteride can promote hair growth effectively while minimizing systemic side effects, particularly those affecting sexual function. A systematic review further supports the efficacy of topical finasteride, revealing substantial decreases in hair loss rates and increases in total and terminal hair counts (Lee 2018). Both scalp and plasma DHT levels were significantly reduced, while serum testosterone levels remained unchanged, highlighting the localized action of topical finasteride with minimal systemic absorption. In another study comparing a novel 0.25% topical finasteride solution to the standard 1 mg oral tablet, both treatments achieved strong and similar inhibition of plasma DHT after 1 week (Caserini 2014). However, the systemic exposure to finasteride was significantly lower with the topical solution, suggesting a reduced risk of systemic side effects. These findings suggest that topical finasteride offers an effective and safer alternative to oral formulations, particularly for patients seeking to minimize systemic risks while achieving meaningful hair restoration outcomes.

Topical Dutasteride

Dutasteride, a dual 5-alpha reductase inhibitor, has emerged as an off-label treatment option for AGA, targeting both type I and type II isoenzymes involved in DHT production. Clinical evidence supports the efficacy of oral dutasteride in promoting hair regrowth. A randomized controlled trial demonstrated that daily administration of 0.5 mg dutasteride significantly increased hair count and width compared to both placebo and finasteride over a 24-week period (Gubelin 2014; Eun 2010). A meta-analysis confirmed its effectiveness in increasing total hair count and improving clinical outcomes, with a comparable safety profile to finasteride (Zhou et al. 2019). Reported side effects, such as decreased libido and erectile dysfunction, are typically mild and reversible upon discontinuation. Although oral dutasteride is well-established, its application as a topical treatment remains under investigation. Due to its large molecular size, direct scalp penetration poses a challenge. However, advanced nanocarrier technologies, including liposomes, transfersomes, and chitosan-coated nanocapsules, have demonstrated the ability to enhance drug delivery to hair follicles. Studies using nanoparticle-based systems have shown effective follicular targeting, increased drug retention in hair shafts, and reduced systemic absorption, suggesting that topical formulations could provide localized benefits with minimized systemic risks (Andrade et al. 2024; Afiune et al. 2020). Further studies are needed to validate the long-term safety and efficacy of these novel approaches, which could expand dutasteride's role in the management of AGA.

Topical Antiandrogens

Topical antiandrogens, such as fluridil and RU58841, are emerging as potential treatments for AGA (Marks et al. 2020). These agents function by locally blocking androgen action on hair follicles, thus avoiding the systemic side effects commonly associated with oral antiandrogens (Sovak et al. 2002). Compound 30a, a highly selective AR antagonist, has demonstrated significant hair-growth-promoting effects in both hair-growth and AGA mouse models (H. Zhang et al. 2024). It showed high skin absorption with minimal systemic exposure, resulting in potent hair growth without detectable toxicity. Comparative studies of topical flutamide and finasteride formulations have shown that both agents significantly increase hair count, length, and diameter in human bald-scalp grafts transplanted onto SCID mice. Flutamide exhibited superior efficacy, producing more hairs per graft and longer hair shafts than finasteride (Sintov et al. 2000). RU58841, a non-steroidal antiandrogen, has displayed efficacy in increasing hair density, thickness, and length in the bald scalp of stump-tailed macaques (Pan et al. 1998). Treated grafts showed higher linear hair growth rates and more active follicles than controls, highlighting its potential as a topical AGA treatment. Fluridil, another promising topical antiandrogen, was evaluated in a clinical study involving AGA patients (Sovak et al. 2002). The study revealed an increase in the anagen percentage from 76% to 85% after 3 months and to 87% after 9 months. Fluridil was well-tolerated, showing no irritation or systemic effects, making it a safe option for managing AGA. Atraric acid, a topical formulation tested in mouse models, demonstrated robust hair regrowth activity (Pulat et al. 2023). AA-TF#15 outperformed minoxidil and oral finasteride, increasing hair regrowth by 58% compared to minoxidil and 41.9% compared to finasteride. These findings suggest its potential as an effective treatment for scalp AGA. Topical antiandrogens represent a promising therapeutic avenue for AGA, offering localized efficacy with minimal systemic exposure. However, larger clinical studies are necessary to validate these findings and optimize their use in hair restoration practices.

Topical Estrogens

Topical estrogen preparations have been explored as potential treatments for female-pattern hair loss. These medications aim to counteract the local effects of androgens on the hair follicles and promote hair growth (Georgala et al. 2004). However, the use of topical estrogens for hair loss is not widely established, and more research is needed to determine their efficacy and optimal formulation.

Ketoconazole

Ketoconazole, an antifungal agent with antiandrogenic and anti-inflammatory properties, has shown promise in managing AGA. By inhibiting 5-alpha reductase, ketoconazole reduces the conversion of testosterone to DHT (Hugo 2004). Additionally, its anti-inflammatory effects help alleviate scalp inflammation, a condition that can exacerbate hair loss (Piérard-Franchimont et al. 1998). Research has demonstrated that ketoconazole improves hair density and increases the proportion of hair follicles in the anagen (growth) phase, with efficacy comparable to minoxidil. It can also be used alongside finasteride to enhance therapeutic outcomes. Ketoconazole is effective not only in individuals with seborrheic dermatitis or dandruff but also in those without these conditions, highlighting its broader application in hair restoration (Piérard-Franchimont et al. 1998). For both men and women with AGA, ketoconazole offers a viable treatment option, either as a standalone therapy or in combination with other treatments, such as topical finasteride. Its dual action of targeting DHT and reducing inflammation provides additional benefits, making it a versatile tool in combating hair loss.

Saw Palmetto

Saw palmetto (*Serenoa repens*) is a herbal supplement believed to inhibit 5-alpha reductase, reducing DHT levels implicated in AGA (Gupta 2022). While some studies suggest it may improve hair density and serve as an alternative for patients hesitant to use conventional therapies like minoxidil and finasteride, clinical evidence remains limited compared to established treatments.

When considering hormonal therapies for hair restoration, practitioners must carefully evaluate the individual patient's hormonal profile, medical history, and treatment goals. It is essential to monitor patients closely for potential side effects and adjust treatment plans accordingly. In some cases, combining hormonal therapies with other hair restoration modalities, such as topical minoxidil or low-level laser therapy, may provide synergistic benefits and optimize treatment outcomes.

Conclusion

Hormonal treatments are integral to the management of hair loss, particularly in cases driven by hormonal imbalances or androgen sensitivity. An understanding of the intricate relationship between hormones and hair growth enables practitioners to develop targeted strategies that address the underlying causes of hair thinning and promote healthier hair growth. The diverse range of hormonal therapies—spanning systemic options such as 5-alpha reductase inhibitors and antiandrogens to topical solutions like finasteride and ketoconazole—allows for personalized treatment plans tailored to each patient's unique hormonal profile and clinical presentation. These therapies not only mitigate the hormonal triggers of hair loss but also offer versatile applications for different patient populations, including men and women with androgenetic alopecia or other hormone-related hair disorders. As research in this field advances, the development of new hormonal treatments and a deeper understanding of hormonal pathways will continue to refine the options available for practitioners and patients.

Chapter 6

Minoxidil

Bilal F. Hamzeh, Haley Guinan, Julyssa A. Renteria and Robert Dorfman

Introduction

Minoxidil is widely recognized as a key first-line therapeutic indicated to treat the most common causes of both male and female alopecia. Available in both topical and oral formulations, minoxidil has versatile clinical utility and plays a crucial role in the clinical management of hair loss. This chapter offers a comprehensive exploration of the versatility, indications, mechanism, and side effects of minoxidil. It also delves into the intricacies of application techniques and strategies for enhancing patient compliance, which is paramount for achieving optimal treatment outcomes. By gaining a deep understanding of the mechanisms of action, efficacy, and practical considerations of both oral and topical minoxidil, practitioners can effectively integrate these options into their hair restoration treatment plans, tailoring them to the unique needs of each patient.

Topical Minoxidil: A Versatile Vasodilator

Minoxidil, a widely recognized and FDA-approved topical treatment for androgenetic alopecia, has become a staple in the management of hair loss for both men and women (Patel et al. 2024). Available over-the-counter as a topical formulation in concentrations of 2% and 5%, with the latter demonstrating superior efficacy, minoxidil has earned its reputation as a reliable, widely used, and accessible option for patients seeking to regain their hair.

The mechanism of action behind minoxidil's efficacy lies in its ability to act as a potassium channel opener, increasing blood flow to the hair follicles, prolonging the anagen phase of the hair growth cycle, and promoting the conversion of miniaturized vellus hairs to more robust terminal hairs. Minoxidil is a prodrug, with the pharmacological benefits being due to its conversion to an active metabolite, minoxidil sulfate, via the enzyme sulfotransferase (Anderson et al. 1998; Gupta et al. 2022).

At the cellular level, minoxidil exerts its effects through several key mechanisms. Firstly, it acts as a vasodilator, dilating the blood vessels surrounding the hair follicles, thereby increasing the delivery of essential nutrients and oxygen to the follicular cells. This enhanced blood flow

DOI: 10.1201/9781032726397-6

creates a more favorable environment for hair growth, nourishing the follicles and supporting their metabolic needs. Secondly, minoxidil has been shown to prolong the anagen phase of the hair cycle, allowing hairs to grow longer and thicker before entering the telogen, or resting, phase. By extending the active growth period, minoxidil enables the production of more substantial and visually impactful hairs. Lastly, this versatile vasodilator stimulates the conversion of vellus hairs, which are fine, short, and often barely visible, into terminal hairs that are thicker, longer, and more pigmented. This transformation is crucial in creating a denser, more aesthetically pleasing head of hair.

The efficacy of minoxidil in promoting hair growth and slowing hair loss has been well established through numerous clinical studies (Chen et al. 2020). A 48-week, placebo-controlled trial investigating the effects of a 5% minoxidil solution applied twice daily revealed a significant increase in hair count and improved patient satisfaction compared to placebo (Olsen et al. 2002). These findings highlight the tangible benefits that minoxidil can provide to patients struggling with hair loss. Furthermore, a comparative study evaluating the effectiveness of 2% and 5% minoxidil concentrations found that the higher concentration yielded significantly better results in stimulating hair growth (Lucky et al. 2004). This evidence underscores the importance of utilizing the most potent formulation available to maximize treatment outcomes.

Minoxidil was initially developed as a medication to treat hypertension but was found to induce hypertrichosis in several patients who were receiving oral minoxidil for over 2 weeks during the progression of the study. Dermatologists were consulted and subsequently assessed the efficacy of topical formulations to observe whether the effect on hair growth could be reproduced. It was soon found that both oral and topical minoxidil could reliably induce significant hair growth without many dose-limiting side effects in patients, and that topical formulations had less of an effect on blood pressure and a more localized effect on hair growth than did oral administration. Minoxidil was soon approved for use both as an antihypertensive agent and as a treatment for alopecia (Zins 1988).

While minoxidil is still used today to treat severe refractory hypertension that has not responded well to other medications, it is more widely used for hair growth. The safety profile of minoxidil is such that it is available in topical formulations over-the-counter in the United States, while oral formulations are available by prescription only due to the higher incidence of side effects from greater systemic exposure to the drug.

Although only approved by the FDA for the treatment of androgenetic alopecia, the efficacy and tolerability of minoxidil have led to extensive exploration in the realms of other forms of alopecia. Ranging from use as monotherapy in scarring alopecia to adjunctive therapy post-hair transplantation, both oral and topical forms of minoxidil have shown promise across the realm of hair restoration and maintenance (Figure 6.1).

Off-label uses of topical minoxidil include:

- *Alopecia areata*: Minoxidil has shown efficacy as a standalone treatment or in combination with other therapies, such as corticosteroids, in producing a positive clinical response (Freire et al. 2019). Alongside two oral JAK inhibitors indicated to treat alopecia areata, minoxidil monotherapy and combination therapy have been investigated in both oral and topical formulations, demonstrating great efficacy in treating alopecia areata. One systematic review evaluating the available literature showed great benefit both in minoxidil monotherapy, administered orally or topically, and in combination with oral JAK inhibitor agents (Raval et al. 2024). As with the use of minoxidil to treat other causes of hair loss, the use of minoxidil to treat alopecia areata is not typically associated with dose-limiting side effects.

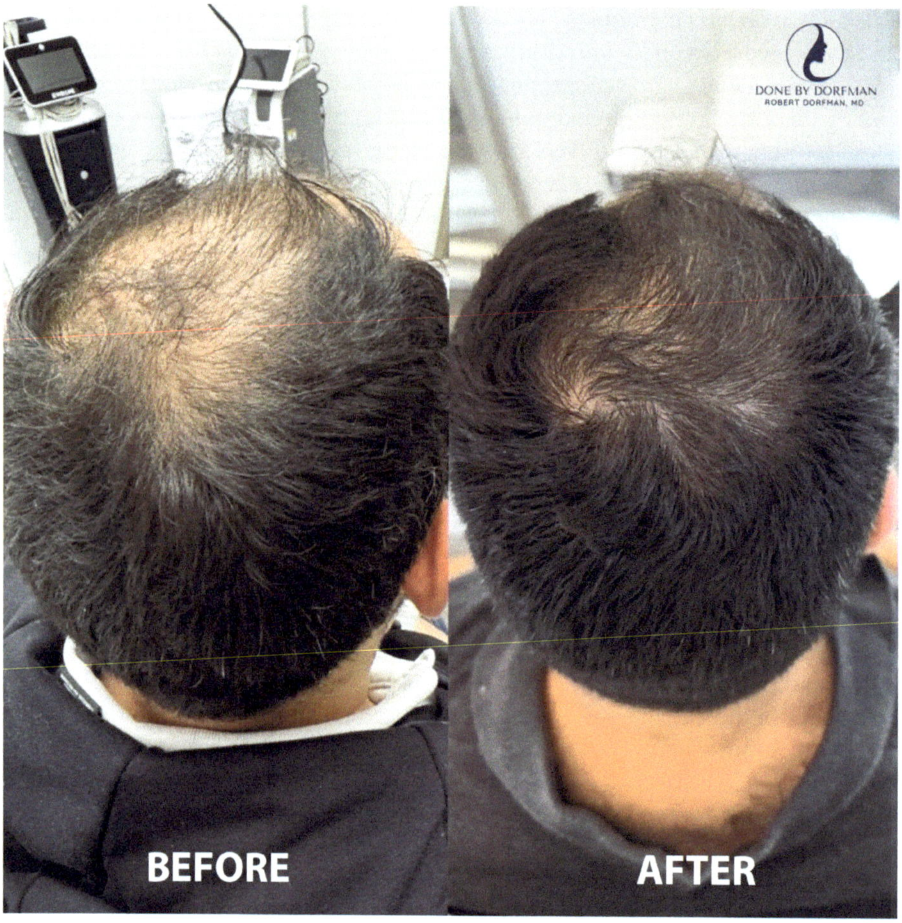

Figure 6.1 Improved hair density in a patient treated with minoxidil monotherapy.

- *Chemotherapy-induced alopecia*: Minoxidil has been effective in reducing hair loss and accelerating hair regrowth in patients undergoing chemotherapy (Duvic et al. 1996). Many chemotherapeutic agents indicated to treat various cancers are also associated with alopecia, with some variability. Doxorubicin-containing chemotherapeutics are often associated with close to total alopecia, while other agents such as fluorouracil, methotrexate, and cyclophosphamide are more often associated with diffuse thinning. Alkylating agents, taxanes, vinca alkaloids, cytotoxic agents, and targeted therapies indicated to treat a wide range of cancers are all associated with alopecia to some degree. Both topical and oral forms of minoxidil have shown promise in helping to treat chemotherapy-induced alopecia, without many side effects of note. Topical formulations can often result in pruritus and scalp irritation, however, which can be addressed by treating patients with low-dose oral minoxidil (Iorizzo et al. 2023).
- *Hair transplant*: Minoxidil can be used before and after hair transplantation to minimize hair loss (telogen effluvium) in patients. However, its use should be paused for 3 days before the transplant to prevent excessive bleeding (Avram et al. 2002). Hair transplantation is often associated with a post-surgical shedding phase and is often expected to require several

months before hair growth can be observed. Moreover, transplanted follicles continue to be susceptible to the same scalp conditions that induce miniaturization and hair loss, meaning steps should be taken to mitigate these conditions and ensure the most optimal conditions for hair growth are maintained. One study utilizing topical minoxidil (3%) found that some patients exhibited regrowth within 2 to 4 weeks post-surgery after initiating minoxidil therapy 48–72 hours after the procedure (Kassimir et al. 1987).

- *Scarring alopecia*: Minoxidil has demonstrated potential antifibrotic effects, making it a possible treatment option during the early stages of dermatoses that lead to scarring alopecia, such as those caused by scalp burns (Ly et al. 2024). Moreover, although scarring alopecia is generally regarded as permanent due to the destruction of hair follicles and the presence of fibrotic changes, separating it from other non-scarring forms of alopecia, minoxidil may still play a role in their treatment. The mainstay of treatment modalities for scarring alopecias is hair transplantation, given the complete loss of hair follicles at the recipient site. Minoxidil has shown benefit as an adjunct alongside hair transplantation in the treatment of scarring alopecias specifically (Tyagi and Singh 2010).
- *Monilethrix*: In this condition, minoxidil helps synchronize hair follicles into the anagen phase, promoting hair growth (Sinclair 2016; Rossi et al. 2011). Monilethrix is an autosomal dominant genetic skin disorder characterized by hair fragility, keratosis, and beading of the hair shaft. Although there is no cure for monilethrix, minoxidil has been shown to reduce hair breakage and fragility, improving appearance by increasing density and length in these patients. Although oral retinoids such as etretinate have been used to reduce hair beading, they show little efficacy in reducing breakage and improving density and length in patients with monilethrix (de Berker and Dawber 1991).
- *Hereditary alopecia or hypotrichosis*: Minoxidil has been effective in thickening hair shafts in cases of hypotrichosis, improving hair density and appearance (Dowd et al. 2019). Hereditary alopecia or hypotrichosis are variable conditions that result in an absence of hair growth—several genes, such as *LIPH*, have been implicated, and the modes of transmission and penetrance are also variable. Minoxidil has been explored as a potential treatment for hereditary alopecia and hypotrichosis. One study found that patients with the *LIPH* autosomal recessive variant improved with topical minoxidil therapy, while a patient with a distinct pathogenic variant, *TRPS1*, did not improve with minoxidil (Taki et al. 2020).

In terms of the practical application of topical minoxidil, proper technique is essential for ensuring optimal absorption and minimizing the risk of side effects. Patients should be instructed to apply the solution or foam directly to the scalp, rather than the hair itself, and to gently massage it in to promote even distribution. Consistency is key, and patients must be advised to use minoxidil twice daily, as directed, to maintain a steady supply of the active ingredient to the hair follicles. It is crucial to emphasize the need for long-term, continuous use, as the benefits of minoxidil may take several months to become apparent. Patients should be informed that the effects of minoxidil are not permanent, and that discontinuation of treatment may lead to a gradual reversal of the achieved hair growth.

Patient compliance is a critical factor in the success of minoxidil therapy, and practitioners must prioritize education and support to ensure that patients adhere to the recommended treatment regimen (Figure 6.2). Consistent application of topical minoxidil for a period of 6–12 months is often required to assess efficacy, which can pose challenges with respect to patient compliance.

Additionally, the first 2 months of minoxidil use in patients can often be accompanied by significant shedding as follicles transition from the telogen to anagen phase, imparting additional

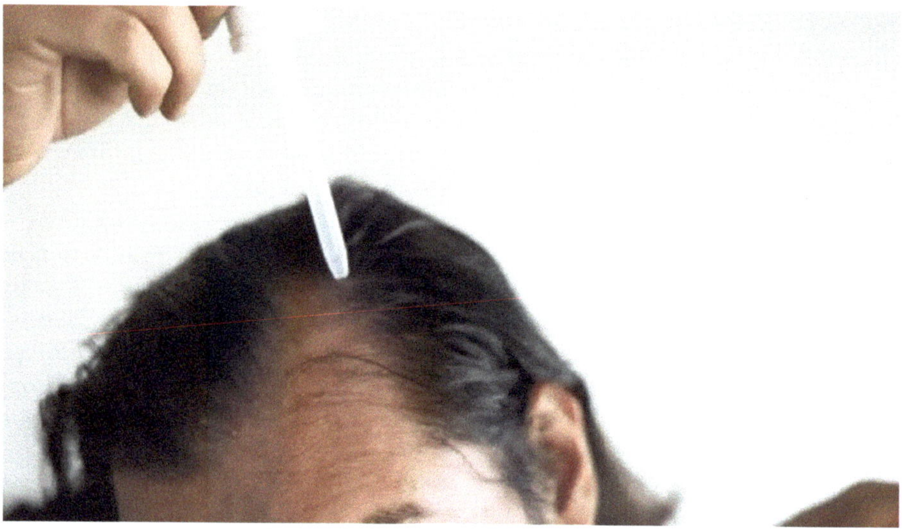

Figure 6.2 **Applying minoxidil (from Shutterstock, under license, https://www.shutterstock.com/video/clip-3529821345-man-applying-minoxidil-hair-dropper-baldness-alopecia).**

challenges with compliance. This period, colloquially referred to as the "dread shed," is expected but can be unsettling for patients, particularly when they are expecting to start a medication that will alleviate their hair loss, not further exacerbate it. This period of increased hair shedding is usually self-limited. A similar shedding period can also often occur when patients transition from topical to oral minoxidil, where one study explored whether maintaining topical minoxidil when initiating low-dose oral minoxidil may help reduce this shedding phase, which it was not found to do (Nohria et al. 2024). Clear communication regarding the importance of consistent, daily use, along with setting realistic expectations about the timeline for visible results, can help foster a strong commitment to the treatment plan. Providing detailed instructions on application techniques and addressing any concerns or side effects promptly can further enhance compliance. Regular follow-up appointments serve as opportunities to monitor progress, assess compliance, and make any necessary adjustments to the treatment approach, ensuring that patients receive the most effective care possible.

Oral Minoxidil: Use Cases and Comparisons

While topical minoxidil has held an uncontested position as the most used hair loss product—owing to wide availability, tolerability, ease of use, and established effect profile—oral formulations of minoxidil do have an important place in a practitioner's toolkit. Primary considerations for the use of oral minoxidil are convenience and patient adherence. Although topical formulations are effective, patients can often struggle with twice-daily applications, undesirable effects on hair texture, and scalp irritation and pruritus (Randolph and Tosti 2021). Data suggests that oral administration of even 1 mg minoxidil daily has a comparable therapeutic effect to twice-daily topical administration of a 5% solution (Asilian et al. 2024; Penha et al. 2024).

The main benefit of oral minoxidil is a more uniform dose, given less variability in the dose consumed orally relative to a topically applied dose. Moreover, as previously discussed, minoxidil is a prodrug requiring the enzyme sulfotransferase to be converted to its active metabolite, minoxidil sulfate. This lends minoxidil metabolism and, by extension, the presence of the active metabolite susceptible to a host of second-order factors that can influence patient response to the drug.

As with any biochemical mediator, the presence of follicular sulfotransferase in the outer root sheath is variable from patient to patient. In fact, sulfotransferase activity in plucked hair follicles has been shown to be a viable predictor of patient response to minoxidil and has been a therapeutic target in non-responders (Roberts et al. 2014). Aspirin has been shown to significantly reduce sulfotransferase activity. In a cohort of 24 subjects, aspirin administration for 2 weeks reduced the percentage predicted to be minoxidil responders from 50% to only 27% (Goren et al. 2018). Conversely, retinoids such as tretinoin have been shown to upregulate sulfotransferase activity and result in an enhanced response to minoxidil. In one study, 43% of subjects initially predicted to be non-responders were converted to responders following 5 days of topical tretinoin application (Sharma et al. 2019).

The regulation of outer root sheath follicular sulfotransferase is dependent on intracellular pH, and recent advances have developed adjuvant topical formulations containing minoxidil and other excipients intended to modulate pH and upregulate minoxidil sulfotransferase (SULT1A1) activity. In one randomized controlled trial, 75% of subjects in the minoxidil plus SULT1A1 adjuvant treatment group compared to 33% of subjects in the minoxidil plus placebo group, with the former group exhibiting more than twice the positive response after 60 days (Dhurat et al. 2021). The highest level of activity of sulfotransferases in humans, however, is in the liver (Pietrauszka and Bergler-Czop, 2020). Although genetic variability does still exert an influence on global sulfotransferase activity, having been shown to predict responsiveness to oral minoxidil in FPHL, the baseline activity of hepatic sulfotransferase is such that oral dosing would still be considered to result in a considerably increased proportion of minoxidil sulfate to minoxidil relative to topical administration (Ramos et al. 2021). As such, given the more uniform dosing, the ease of administration and resultant improved patient adherence, and the higher activity of hepatic relative to follicular sulfotransferases, oral minoxidil is a preferred route of administration in many cases.

Along with the ability to treat a wide variety of alopecias, minoxidil has been an important adjunct post-hair transplant along with other medications such as finasteride. Unlike finasteride, minoxidil is not generally considered to be a must-have post-transplant medication, but the benefits of improving scalp blood flow and upregulating chemical mediators that have a positive effect on the hair cycle make it a favorable option alongside finasteride. Oral minoxidil at doses of 2.5 to 5 mg once daily for men or 1.25 to 2.5 mg once daily for women, is often preferred alongside finasteride post-hair transplant for several reasons. Among them, oral dosing negates the possibility of local irritation and pruritus, which is particularly detrimental post-hair transplant. Moreover, oral dosing subjects minoxidil to first-pass hepatic metabolism, likely converting more of the drug to its active metabolite relative to topical administration as discussed earlier.

The Art and Science of Application

The success of topical hair loss treatments hinges not only on the selection of the appropriate medication but also on the mastery of proper application techniques and the cultivation of patient compliance. Practitioners must recognize that the manner in which topical treatments are applied can significantly influence their absorption, distribution, and ultimate effectiveness. By providing clear, detailed instructions on application methods and emphasizing the importance of consistent, long-term use, practitioners can empower their patients to optimize the benefits of their topical treatment regimens.

Before applying any topical treatment, patients should be advised to thoroughly cleanse their scalp with a gentle, non-medicated shampoo or conditioner, and allow it to dry completely. This preparatory step serves to remove any dirt, oil, or styling products that may interfere with the absorption of the active ingredients, ensuring that the treatment can penetrate the scalp effectively. Once the scalp is clean and dry, patients should be instructed to part their hair and apply the topical treatment directly to the affected areas of the scalp, rather than the hair itself. This targeted application approach maximizes the concentration of the medication at the site of action, promoting optimal efficacy. Patients should then gently massage the product into the scalp, using circular motions to distribute it evenly and facilitate absorption. This gentle massage also helps to stimulate blood flow to the hair follicles, further enhancing the delivery of nutrients and oxygen necessary for healthy hair growth.

Dosage and frequency of application are critical factors in the success of topical hair loss treatments, and practitioners must provide clear guidelines to their patients. Each topical medication has its own recommended dosage and application schedule, which have been carefully determined through clinical studies to balance efficacy and safety. For 5% aerosol minoxidil, the recommended dosage is half a capful twice daily for men and once daily for women. The 2% topical minoxidil solution has a recommended dosage of 1 mL twice daily for women. The dosage recommendation for 2% and 5% topical minoxidil is 1 mL twice daily for men. Patients should be advised to adhere strictly to these guidelines, applying the prescribed amount of product at the specified intervals. Consistency is key, as sporadic or inconsistent use may compromise the effectiveness of the treatment and lead to suboptimal results. Practitioners should also discuss the optimal timing for applying topical treatments, such as allowing sufficient time for absorption before bedtime or before styling the hair, to ensure that the product remains in contact with the scalp for the necessary duration. Additionally, patients should be counseled on any precautions associated with treatment, such as avoiding contact with the eyes or washing hands thoroughly after application, to minimize the risk of adverse effects.

Patient compliance is a critical determinant of the success of topical hair loss treatments, and practitioners must prioritize education and motivation to foster adherence. Patients should be informed that visible results may take several months to manifest, as the hair follicles require time to respond to the treatment and initiate the regrowth process. This understanding helps to manage expectations and maintain patient commitment, even in the absence of immediate gratification. Practitioners should emphasize the importance of consistent, daily use and the need for long-term perseverance to achieve and maintain the desired outcomes. By setting realistic goals and conveying the potential for slowing further hair loss and promoting gradual regrowth, rather than promising a complete reversal of baldness, practitioners can help patients develop a realistic and sustainable approach to their hair restoration journey.

Addressing potential side effects and providing strategies for their management is another crucial aspect of promoting patient compliance. While topical hair loss treatments are generally well-tolerated, some patients may experience local irritation, itching, or redness at the site of application. Practitioners should encourage patients to report any persistent or bothersome side effects promptly, allowing for timely intervention and adjustment of the treatment plan if necessary. By proactively discussing these concerns and offering solutions, such as reducing the frequency of application or switching to a different formulation, practitioners can minimize the impact of side effects on patient adherence and overall treatment success.

Regular follow-up appointments are essential for monitoring treatment response, reinforcing compliance, and providing ongoing support to patients. These visits serve as opportunities to assess the progress of hair growth, evaluate the effectiveness of the current treatment regimen, and make any necessary adjustments. By engaging in open, supportive dialogue with patients, practitioners can identify and address any challenges or barriers to adherence, offering guidance and encouragement to help patients stay committed to their hair restoration goals. Celebrating milestones and acknowledging the patient's efforts can further bolster motivation and foster a strong therapeutic alliance, ultimately enhancing the likelihood of successful treatment outcomes.

Microneedling

Microneedling, also called dermarolling or percutaneous collagen induction (PCI), is a minimally invasive treatment for hair loss that involves the use of at-home devices, either manual or electric and often drum-shaped (for manual dermarolling) or pen-shaped (for electric dermarolling) with fine needles that puncture the stratum corneum and create controlled micro-injuries to the scalp, promoting hair growth by stimulating the wound healing response, increasing blood flow to the area, and inducing the release of growth factors that foster a favorable environment for hair growth (Fertig et al. 2018). This upregulation of the inflammatory response, inducing neovascularization and collagen production, stimulates hair growth through a mechanism similar to that of laser therapies and other inflammation-inducing modalities.

Microneedling is often performed adjunctively with topical treatments for hair loss, particularly with topical minoxidil, because of this synergistic effect—both microneedling and minoxidil are thought to promote hair growth via increasing blood flow and upregulating growth factors such as PDGF, VEGF, and TGF-beta, inducing angiogenesis and increased hair growth. One study showed that microneedling monotherapy was more effective than topical minoxidil monotherapy in increasing total hair count, and found that microneedling and topical minoxidil combination therapy was significantly more effective in increasing total hair count when compared to monotherapies alone (Gupta et al. 2022). Like other modalities such as light and ultrasound therapy, microneedling may also synergize with topical treatments such as minoxidil by improving transdermal drug delivery.

Microneedling has thus become an important adjunct in the non-surgical management of hair loss both due to the efficacy, the synergy with other pharmacotherapeutic treatment modalities, and the accessibility. Devices are easily accessible to patients and can be used routinely alongside their topical treatments (Figure 6.3). Microneedling is not without risks. It can be associated with erythema, pain, post-inflammatory hyperpigmentation, dry skin, and irritant contact dermatitis in addition to more serious reactions such as tram-track scarring and granulomatous reactions (S. Chu et al. 2021). Although minimally invasive, microneedling is a modality in which microabrasions are produced on the scalp, which can make patients susceptible to infection. Proper counseling on the routine sterilization of devices, often with alcohol, is crucial in cases where the patient and provider agree that microneedling will be pursued as a beneficial adjunct to their treatment.

Scalp micropigmentation (SMP) is a procedure that also involves microneedling but utilizes pigmentation akin to tattooing that is used to conceal areas of low hair density. It offers a permanent concealer for areas of lower hair density, creating the illusion of increased density by applying pigmented dots on the scalp between pores. The procedure requires considerable artistic acumen, necessitating the impregnation of pigment into the upper dermis (Rassman et al. 2015) (Figure 6.4).

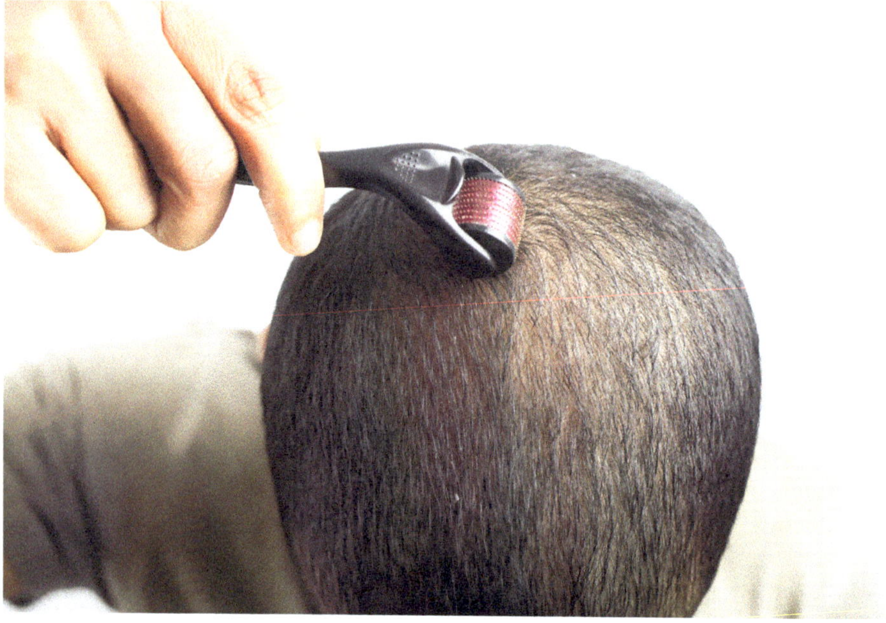

Figure 6.3 Collagen induction therapy using microneedling (from Shutterstock, under license).

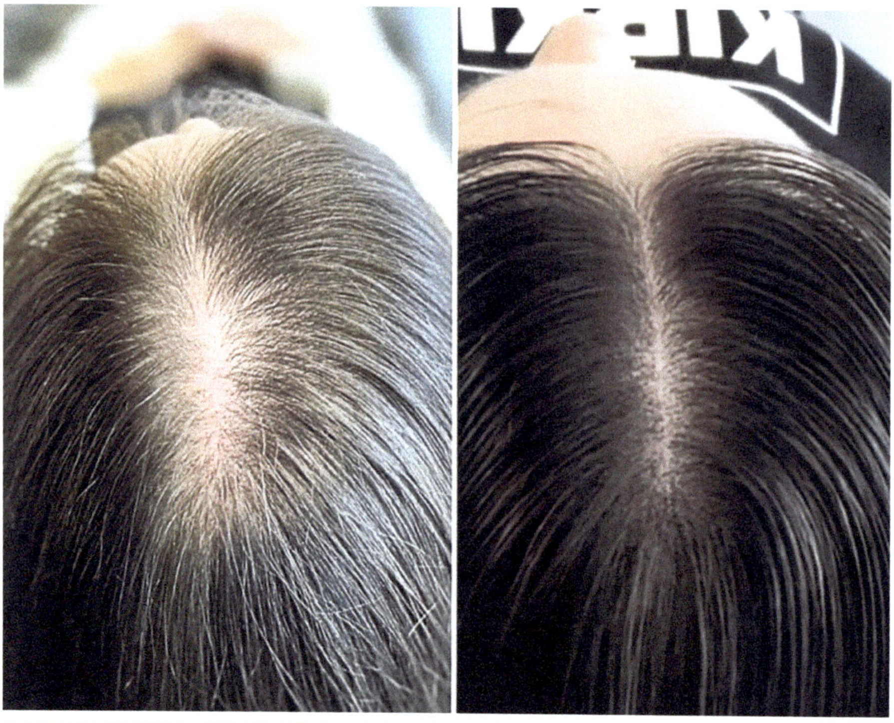

Figure 6.4 Improved appearance of hair density in a patient who underwent scalp micropigmentation (SMP).

Side Effects and Contraindications

Although minoxidil is generally very well tolerated, as reflected in its availability over-the-counter without a prescription in the United States and many other countries, and in the prevalence of prescriptions for oral formulations, it is not without side effects, including some rare but serious adverse drug reactions. As previously described, topical minoxidil is associated with many side effects relating to the active agent, minoxidil, or one of the many excipients used in the foam and liquid formulations. Among these side effects, pruritus and general irritation of the area of application are the most common.

Hypertrichosis is a side effect commonly observed in both oral and topical forms of minoxidil, as can be expected. Hypertrichosis is among the most common dose-limiting side effects of minoxidil use and is reportedly seen more commonly in female patients than in male patients, in addition to being more frequently reported as a side effect of oral minoxidil compared to topical minoxidil (Dawber and Rundegren 2003). The hypertrichotic effect of minoxidil at sites other than the scalp, mainly the face, is reversible and does not always require cessation of minoxidil therapy.

Given minoxidil was initially developed as an antihypertensive medication, the primary non-dermatological side effects of minoxidil are related to the circulatory system. Most prevalent among these side effects are increased fluid retention due to increased retention of sodium, a complication noted during the initial clinical trials of minoxidil as an antihypertensive, originally negated with loop diuretics. Other hypotensive symptoms, such as lightheadedness, transient postural dizziness, palpitations, and reflex tachycardia, are associated with minoxidil use, occurring more frequently with oral minoxidil due to the increased systemic exposure to the drug relative to topical formulations. Rare but serious circulatory side effects, such as ECG abnormalities and pericardial effusion, are associated with the use of oral minoxidil. One report details the case of a previously healthy female patient who developed pericardial effusion at a dosage of 1.25 mg of minoxidil orally after being admitted with concerns of shortness of breath, lower limb edema, and orthopnea (Trüeb et al. 2022). The package insert of oral minoxidil marketed for the treatment of arterial hypertension at doses of 2.5 and 10 mg, Loniten, does list pericardial effusion as an adverse effect with a frequency of 3% to 5%. Outside of dermatological and cardiological/circulatory side effects, minoxidil has also been associated with psychiatric side effects such as depression.

Relative to topical formulations of minoxidil, oral formulations have an increased incidence of side effects including diffuse hypertrichosis, or increased hair growth in unwanted areas, circulatory issues such as edema, and hypotensive symptoms including dizziness and headaches, all owing to an increase in systemic exposure to minoxidil from oral administration. Nascimento et al. (2020) list the results. The highest reported incidences of side effects are up to 93% hypertrichosis (reported by Lueangarun et al. 2015), 25% acne (Wambier et al. 2019), 10% ECG abnormalities (Lueangarun et al. 2015), 5.5% dizziness (Perera and Sinclair 2017), 4.8% limb edema (Jimenez-Cauhe et al. 2019), 2.4% hair shedding (Jimenez-Caube et al. 2017), 2% hypotensive symptoms (Sinclair 2018), and 2% urticaria (Sinclair 2018). See Figure 6.5.

Contraindications for the use of minoxidil are few and generally depend on the case-by-case judgment of the practitioner. One such contraindication is pregnancy and breastfeeding; although minoxidil has not been associated with any teratogenic effects, the transmission of the drug to a developing embryo or to infants via breast milk has not been thoroughly characterized and warrants caution (Suchonwanit et al. 2019). Patients with severe uncontrolled hypotension or hypertension being managed with other medications should be assessed for candidacy on a case-by-case basis; for example, concomitant use of guanethidine, an antihypertensive, with minoxidil can

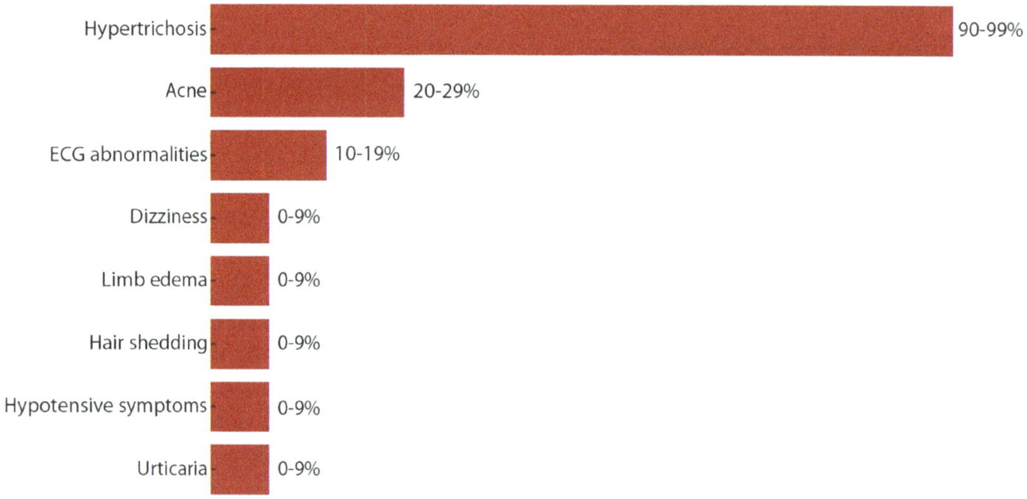

Figure 6.5 Frequency (%) of reported adverse effects associated with the use of minoxidil.

cause severe hypotension (Mutterperl et al. 1976). Other medications can also have an impact on the efficacy of minoxidil: cyclosporine can exacerbate the hypertrichotic side effects of minoxidil (Sever et al. 1990), while aspirin, as previously discussed, can reduce the efficacy of topical minoxidil by downregulating the activity of sulfotransferases (Goren et al. 2018).

Conclusion

Like with all treatments indicated for hair loss, practitioners can observe a range of efficacy among patients based on underlying alopecia etiology, individual physiology, patient adherence, and the presence of side effects. For patients struggling with adherence to topical minoxidil, oral formulations should be considered after patients are counseled on the potential increased incidence of side effects. The art of successful topical treatment lies not only in the selection of the appropriate medication but also in the mastery of application techniques and the cultivation of patient compliance. Through clear instruction, patient education, and ongoing support, practitioners can empower their patients to optimize the benefits of topical hair loss treatments, leading to more satisfying and enduring results.

For both oral and topical formulations, minoxidil can induce a shedding period, colloquially referred to as the "dread shed," that can have a negative effect on patient adherence (Nohria et al. 2024). Patients should be counseled on the possibility of a minoxidil-induced shedding phase beginning 2–4 weeks after initiating treatment, lasting 3–6 weeks.

In terms of long-term efficacy, minoxidil helps patients maintain non-vellus hair regrowth over several years, dependent on patient adherence to the treatment plan (Olsen et al. 1987). Clinical monitoring of hair loss progression is vital, as the long-term mitigation of hair loss with minoxidil-only regimens is variable and may require the eventual addition of other therapies such as 5-alpha reductase inhibitors.

Owing to its tolerability, efficacy, versatility, and reputation, minoxidil has been and will likely continue to be among the most important tools in a practitioner's arsenal against hair loss.

Chapter 7

Finasteride and the 5-Alpha Reductase Inhibitors

Bilal F. Hamzeh, Haley Guinan, Julyssa A. Renteria and Robert Dorfman

Finasteride and the Battle Against DHT

Finasteride, a medication belonging to the class of 5-alpha reductase inhibitors (5ARIs), has emerged as a powerful tool in the fight against androgenetic alopecia, particularly in men (though it also plays a role in the treatment of postmenopausal women). FDA-approved for the treatment of male-pattern baldness, finasteride works by targeting the root cause of this common form of hair loss: dihydrotestosterone (DHT). By inhibiting the conversion of testosterone to DHT, a potent androgen that plays a pivotal role in the miniaturization of hair follicles, finasteride helps to slow the progression of hair loss and promote the regrowth of healthier, thicker hairs.

The mechanism of action behind finasteride's effectiveness lies in its ability to selectively inhibit the enzyme 5-alpha reductase type II, which is responsible for catalyzing the conversion of testosterone to DHT in the hair follicles. By blocking this critical step in the androgen pathway, finasteride significantly reduces the levels of DHT in the scalp, thereby minimizing its detrimental effects on hair follicles. This reduction of DHT levels limits the miniaturizing influence of the androgen on hair follicles, enabling them to produce thicker, more robust hairs less susceptible to shedding and thinning.

The efficacy of finasteride in treating androgenetic alopecia has been extensively documented in numerous clinical trials. A landmark 2-year study involving men with male-pattern baldness demonstrated that a daily dose of 1 mg finasteride resulted in a significant increase in hair count, improved scalp coverage, and a notable reduction in the progression of hair loss compared to placebo (Kaufman et al. 1998). These findings underscore the potent impact that finasteride can have on reversing the course of androgenetic alopecia and restoring a fuller, more youthful head of hair. Long-term studies have further confirmed that the benefits of finasteride can be sustained with continued use, providing patients with a reliable and effective solution for managing their hair loss over an extended period (Rossi et al. 2011) (Figure 7.1).

DOI: 10.1201/9781032726397-7

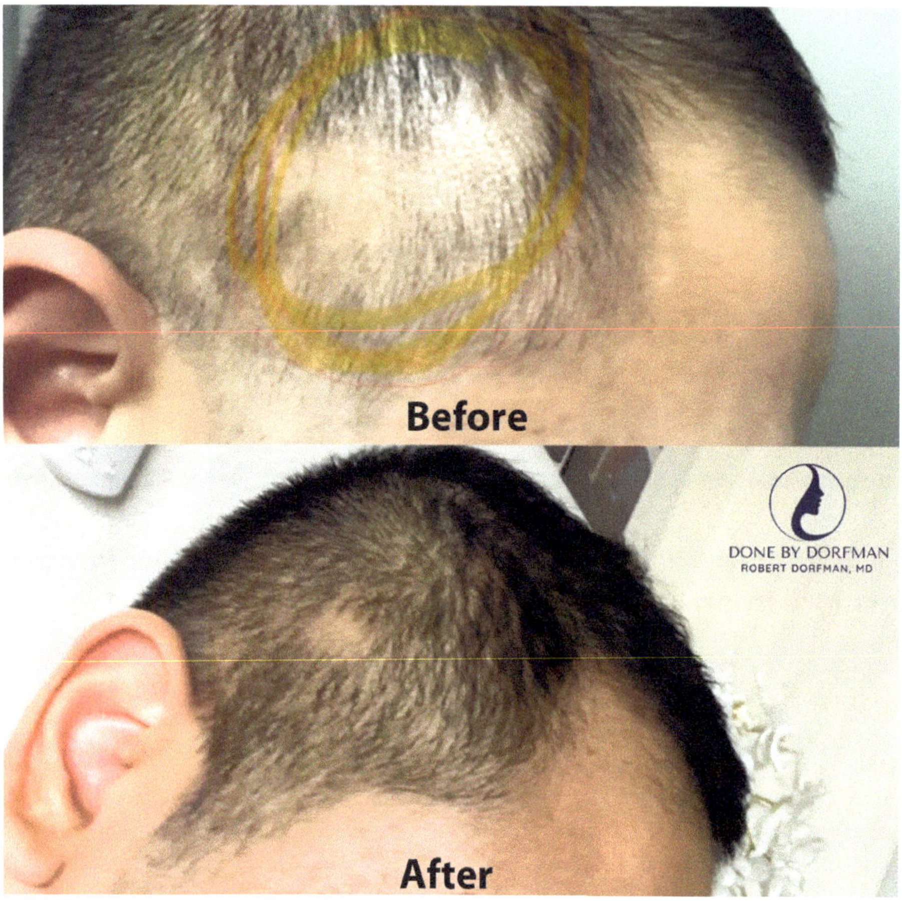

Figure 7.1 Before and after images demonstrating the impact of 5-alpha reductase inhibitors, such as finasteride and dutasteride, on androgenetic alopecia (AGA). (Top) Areas of significant hair thinning and miniaturization of hair follicles. (Bottom) Following sustained treatment, visible hair regrowth and increased hair density.

When it comes to the administration of finasteride, the standard dosage is 1 mg taken orally once daily, though the dosage may be increased to up to 5 mg daily depending on the patient's tolerance and side effect profile. Patients should be advised to take the medication at the same time each day to maintain consistent drug levels in the body and optimize treatment outcomes. It is important to set realistic expectations with patients, emphasizing that the visible benefits of finasteride may take several months to become apparent, as the hair follicles require time to adjust to the altered hormonal environment and initiate the regrowth process. Patients should be counseled on the necessity of continuous, long-term use to maintain the achieved results, as discontinuation of finasteride may lead to a gradual reversal of hair growth and a return to the previous state of hair loss.

Finasteride is also available for use as a topical spray, sometimes in combination with minoxidil. The benefits and drawbacks of topical finasteride relative to oral finasteride are similar to those discussed with minoxidil. Topical administration, while posing adherence problems and some dermatological side effects relating to hair texture and scalp discomfort, does offer the benefit of less systemic exposure to the medication. Topical finasteride is associated with a lower incidence of side effects related to reduced serum DHT concentrations, while maintaining similar efficacy. (Piraccini et al. 2022).

Ensuring patient compliance with finasteride therapy is crucial for achieving and sustaining optimal hair growth. Practitioners should devote ample time to educating patients on the importance of daily, consistent use, and the need for long-term commitment to the treatment plan. Setting realistic expectations regarding the timeline for visible improvements and the extent of hair regrowth that can be achieved is essential for maintaining patient motivation and adherence. Open and honest discussions about potential side effects, such as sexual dysfunction, and providing strategies for managing these concerns can further enhance compliance. Regular follow-up appointments serve as opportunities to assess treatment response, monitor for adverse effects, and reinforce the importance of consistent use, fostering a strong therapeutic alliance between the practitioner and the patient.

Oral Finasteride: Use Cases and Comparisons

While oral finasteride is the only formulation approved by the FDA for the treatment of androgenetic alopecia, topical formulations have gained popularity, either as monotherapies or in combination with minoxidil. The benefit of topical use of finasteride lies in the reduced systemic exposure to the drug, resulting in a reduced probability of side effects relative to oral formulations. As DHT plays an important role in sexual function, particularly in male patients, reduced serum DHT concentrations resulting from systemic exposure to finasteride may result in sexual side effects that can be mitigated through the use of topical formulations.

One phase III randomized controlled trial found that the incidence of sexual side effects was 2.8% in patients receiving topical finasteride, compared to 3.3% receiving placebo and 4.8% receiving oral finasteride, corresponding to a reduction relative to baseline in serum DHT of 34.6% in the topical finasteride group compared to 55.6% in the oral finasteride group (Piraccini et al. 2022). Given the efficacy of topical finasteride has been shown to be similar to that of oral finasteride, it can be considered an option for patients concerned about side effects from oral use or in patients actively experiencing side effects.

The Art and Science of Application

As with minoxidil, the topical application of finasteride requires consistency and sound application technique. The scalp should be cleansed prior to application in order to remove dirt and oils and allow maximum exposure of the scalp to the applied solution. Finasteride is typically available topically at a strength between 0.1% and 0.25% (w/w), with the clinical trial previously mentioned assessing the efficacy of a 0.25% (w/w) solution. The topical spray is usually applied over affected areas in the morning after cleansing the scalp and left on for the remainder of the day (roughly 8 hours) before being washed off in the evening. Depending on patient preference, it can also be applied in the evening and left overnight during sleep to be rinsed off in the morning.

As with any topical medications, finasteride and the excipients used in topical formulations may result in scalp irritation and pruritus. It is important to discuss concerns pertaining to discomfort resulting from the use of topical finasteride with patients and counsel on the importance of consistent use. Concerns and challenges pertaining to topical administration of minoxidil generally apply to topical finasteride. Both due to the improved patient adherence to oral medications and the wider availability of oral finasteride relative to newer topical formulations, oral finasteride is often preferred over topical, except in cases where a patient expresses concerns about side effects related to systemic absorption of the drug.

Side Effects and Contraindications

The side effects of finasteride use, although generally uncommon, are of greater concern to patients than those associated with minoxidil and are more likely to be dose-limiting or require cessation of treatment. Side effects from finasteride use are thought primarily to occur secondary to its effect on serum DHT levels; by inhibiting 5-alpha reductase, finasteride significantly reduces serum DHT levels in patients. This can result primarily in sexual side effects ranging from erectile dysfunction and ejaculation issues to low libido, in addition to psychiatric side effects such as depression and anxiety. Finasteride has also been associated with persistent gynecomastia. Moreover, the use of finasteride has been associated with a condition termed "post-finasteride syndrome," a constellation of psychiatric, sexual, and neurological symptoms occurring during finasteride therapy and persisting after cessation of the drug, analogous to post-SSRI syndromes described in the literature.

The sexual side effects of finasteride are of primary concern to patients and have been documented to occur in anywhere from 0.9% to 38% of patients (Traish et al. 2015; Erdemir et al. 2008). The effect on erectile function has been postulated to occur secondary to reduced activity of nitric oxide synthase due to reduced circulating DHT, but the exact mechanism remains unclear. Several studies have shown an increased rate of erectile dysfunction, ejaculatory dysfunction, and reduced libido in patients taking finasteride relative to placebo. These are generally accepted as rare but well-established side effects of finasteride use (Hirshburg et al. 2016). If sexual side effects do occur with finasteride use, there is evidence that the severity of symptoms does improve over the course of treatment and can often return to a rate similar to that of placebo (Stoner 1994). One study found that, on average, the occurrence of sexual side effects associated with finasteride use began 1.8 years following the start of therapy and persisted for 5 months after stopping the medication (Ali et al. 2015).

An increasingly controversial topic is that of persistent side effects resulting from finasteride use. A constellation of symptoms, including neurological issues such as brain fog; psychiatric issues such as anhedonia, depression, and anxiety; and, chiefly, sexual issues such as erectile dysfunction and low libido persist after discontinuing finasteride. Post-finasteride syndrome (PFS) is controversial in the medical field as there is a paucity of blinded studies evaluating the credibility of the claims of permanent side effects, with some arguing the syndrome to be, in large part, psychosomatic and that associations identified in the literature may be spurious as they are confounded by significant selection bias (Singh and Avram 2014). One pharmacoepidemiological study found a strong association between low-dose finasteride use in young men, resulting in more expected reporting of sexual dysfunction than any other drug evaluated. Finasteride use was found to be associated with sexual dysfunction and suicidal ideation in the retrospectively evaluated cohort, with six fatal cases reported (Ali et al. 2015).

Psychiatric side effects such as depression and anxiety are associated with use of oral finasteride. In fact, the package insert for Propecia (brand name of finasteride) includes depression as a possible adverse effect. Although generally rare, it is important to counsel patients on the possibility of psychiatric side effects associated with finasteride use and to foster a relationship in which patients feel comfortable evaluating any progression of symptoms and engaging in open discussion with their practitioners. One study found that in a mixed cohort of both male and female patients, moderate to severe depression developed in 19 out of 23 patients on a course of 1 mg finasteride daily (oral). Depression was reported to affect social relationships, eating and sleeping behaviors, and was associated with anxiety in some patients. Symptoms resolved promptly in all patients after cessation of the drug, and quickly relapsed in two patients who re-initiated finasteride therapy (Altomare and Capella 2002). Irwig (2012) showed not only a significant increase in depressive symptoms in former users of finasteride relative to the control group (75% vs. 10%, $P < 0.0001$) but also a significantly increased rate of suicidal ideation in the finasteride group (44% vs. 3%, $P < 0.0001$) (Irwig 2012). Like the sexual side effects of finasteride use, the psychiatric side effects are not well understood and are thought to result from dysregulation of androgen signaling, though further research is required to further characterize the nature and mechanism of these side effects.

Gynecomastia is also a well-documented side effect of high-dose finasteride use and is not unexpected given the mechanism of action of finasteride. Finasteride use in benign prostatic hyperplasia, for example, was associated with a twofold greater risk of causing gynecomastia relative to placebo after treatment for 6 months (Fang et al. 2019). However, low-dose finasteride, indicated to treat androgenetic alopecia, is also associated with the development of persistent gynecomastia. One report details the case of a 20-year-old man taking 1 mg of finasteride orally once daily who developed bilateral gynecomastia confirmed radiologically. Finasteride was discontinued, and raloxifene, a selective estrogen receptor modulator, was initiated at 60 mg/day but was unsuccessful in yielding a satisfactory reduction in the gynecomastia. The patient subsequently underwent bilateral mammoplasty, which revealed the presence of glandular breast tissue (Farkas et al. 2024).

Like minoxidil, finasteride has few absolute contraindications, with patient candidacy being determined on a case-by-case basis. Among the few contraindications are pregnancy and breastfeeding in female patients, in addition to pediatric patients. Due to the effect of finasteride on androgens and the lack of safety established in pediatric patients, finasteride is not approved for use in this population.

Finasteride and Prostate Cancer

Beyond the effect on male hair growth, finasteride has also been shown to have an effect on the development of prostate cancer in male patients due to its antiandrogenic mechanism of action. In the Prostate Cancer Prevention Trial (PCPT), finasteride was shown to reduce the relative risk of prostate cancer by 24.8%, but did show an increase in high-grade prostate cancer of 26.9% (Thompson et al. 2003), although more recent studies have shown no significant differences in survival between finasteride-treated men and placebo group (Thompson et al. 2013). Further studies have also demonstrated that bias may have accounted for the increased risk of aggressive prostate cancers in the finasteride-treated group, and that finasteride may not actually pose this risk (Redman et al. 2008). Nonetheless, this concern regarding the potential increased risk of developing aggressive prostate cancers in men treated with finasteride has effectively eliminated the use of finasteride in prostate cancer prevention. By virtue of its 5ARI mechanism of action, finasteride can also reduce prostate volume and decrease levels of prostate-specific antigen (PSA), a biomarker useful in the detection of prostate cancer. Studies have shown that finasteride can result in a reduction of PSA of up to 50% during the first year of treatment (Etzioni et al. 2005), with an adjustment factor of 2–2.5 being required to interpret serum PSA accurately (Guess et al. 1996). Other studies have shown a similar effect of dutasteride on reducing prostate volume and PSA, even demonstrating a more significant reduction in the dutasteride-treated group relative to the finasteride-treated group (Choi et al. 2010). As such, it is crucial that practitioners prescribing any 5ARIs account for these reductions in PSA during treatment and ensure that patients notify other providers, such as urologists who may be managing prostate health, of treatment with 5ARIs.

Other 5-Alpha Reductase Inhibitors

In addition to finasteride, other DHT blockers have emerged as potential options for the treatment of androgenetic alopecia. Dutasteride, an oral 5-alpha reductase inhibitor that blocks both type I and type II enzymes, has shown promise in clinical studies, potentially offering greater efficacy (Zhou 2019) than finasteride (Olsen et al. 2006). However, it is important to note that dutasteride is not currently FDA approved for the treatment of hair loss, and its use for this indication is considered off-label. Topical formulations of finasteride have also been developed, aiming to minimize systemic absorption and reduce the risk of side effects associated with oral administration. While not yet FDA-approved, studies have yielded encouraging results in terms of hair growth promotion and reduced systemic exposure compared to oral finasteride (Caserini et al. 2014).

Unlike finasteride, which only inhibits type 2 5-alpha reductase, dutasteride inhibits type 1 and 2 isoenzymes of 5-alpha reductase (Nickel et al. 2004). Results of a double-blind phase II trial show significant differences in the inhibition of DHT when comparing dutasteride and finasteride; relative to a 5 mg oral dose of finasteride, a daily oral dose of 0.5 mg dutasteride resulted in significantly reduced DHT levels compared to baseline (94.7 $\pm$ 3.3% vs. 70.8 $\pm$ 18.3%, $P < 0.001$) (Clark et al. 2004). It is still unclear, however, whether a selective versus dual inhibition of 5-alpha reductase results in a clinically significant difference in finasteride versus dutasteride therapy. Outside of the variable pharmacodynamic profile, dutasteride also possesses a markedly increased half-life relative to finasteride; the half-life of finasteride is only 6–8 hours, generally requiring daily oral dosing, dutasteride has a half-life of 4–5 weeks, meaning the drug can be administered less frequently than finasteride (Gisleskog et al. 1999). For example, I frequently prescribe dutasteride at 0.5 mg twice weekly or every 3 days, compared with finasteride that is typically prescribed to be taken daily.

Outside of pharmacodynamic and pharmacokinetic differences, oral dutasteride shows a similar occurrence of side effects when compared with oral finasteride, owing to the similar effect on serum DHT concentrations. One retrospective study found a rate of side effects of 2.6% in a cohort of 307 patients requiring discontinuation of the drug. These side effects included from low libido (n = 4), gynecomastia (n = 2), mood disorder (n = 1), and erectile dysfunction (n = 1) (Vañó-Galván et al. 2020). Like finasteride, topical dutasteride has also been explored as a potential alternative to oral dutasteride. One randomized controlled trial assessed the efficacy of microneedling alone versus microneedling plus topical 0.01% dutasteride and found markedly improved growth in the dutasteride (52.9% in the microneedling plus dutasteride group vs. 17.6% in the microneedling plus saline group, P = 0.037) (Sánchez-Meza et al. 2022). Preliminary data, however, have shown that topical dutasteride may not be as effective as oral dutasteride in increasing mean hair count (Herz-Ruelas et al. 2020). The efficacy of topical dutasteride may be limited by molecular size, which affects the ability of the compound to effectively penetrate the skin and inhibit 5-alpha reductase. As such, supporting data are limited when compared with topical finasteride. Intralesional dutasteride microinjections have also been explored as a novel and promising alternative to both oral and topical formulations, yielding improved hair growth and reduced hair loss with a lower incidence of side effects, including sexual side effects (Saceda-Corralo et al. 2022).

In addition to the 5-alpha reductase inhibitors, ketoconazole, an antifungal agent with antiandrogenic properties, has also demonstrated some benefits in reducing scalp inflammation and complementing other hair loss treatments when used in shampoo form (Fields et al. 2020). Long-term use of topical ketoconazole at a strength of 2% has been shown to increase the density, size, and proportion of anagen follicles (Piérard-Franchimont et al. 1998). The mechanism of action of ketoconazole lies in its inhibition of cytochrome P450 and resultant degradation of steroid precursors, including DHT (Hugo Perez 2004). As such, ketoconazole is a valuable adjunctive treatment for androgenetic alopecia alongside 5-alpha reductase inhibitors and minoxidil, and is frequently prescribed to be used alongside these agents. I frequently recommend the use of ketoconazole shampoos, availablc both over-the-counter and by prescription, to augment other treatments for androgenetic alopecia.

5-Alpha Reductase Inhibitors in Female-Pattern Alopecia

Minoxidil remains the first-line treatment for female-pattern alopecia; however, the utilization of 5ARIs such as finasteride and dutasteride is increasing. It is important to have a thorough discussion with your patient about their plans to conceive, as the use of 5ARIs can pose significant risks during pregnancy. Properly assessing their reproductive plans is crucial to prevent potential harm, such as birth defects, associated with 5ARIs.

The primary concern with 5ARIs in women who are pregnant or may become pregnant is the elevated risk of teratogenic effects, specifically congenital malformations in male fetuses, as has been evidenced in animal studies (Bowman et al. 2003). Exposure to 5ARIs during pregnancy has been associated with an increased incidence of abnormal development of male external genitalia, including hypospadias observed in rhesus monkeys (Prahalada et al. 1997). Consequently, 5ARIs are classified as pregnancy category X and are contraindicated during pregnancy. Some authorities recommend pregnancy testing prior to initiating 5ARI therapy and emphasize the importance of concurrent use of reliable contraception in nonpregnant women of reproductive potential (Hirshburg 2016). However, these medications can be beneficial in postmenopausal females.

5ARIs are still beneficial in women experiencing hair loss because androgens such as DHT play a fundamental role in female physiology as they do in male physiology. As women have circulating testosterone that is converted to DHT via 5-alpha reductase isoenzymes that can have a deleterious impact on hair growth, 5ARIs can play a crucial role in the treatment of female-pattern hair loss. Although studies evaluating the efficacy of 5ARIs on female-pattern alopecia are limited due to the teratogenicity of these agents, there is some literature demonstrating their efficacy. Finasteride has been shown to increase hair density and reduce hair shedding in pre- and post-menopausal women with or without hyperandrogenism (Iamsumang et al. 2020). Dutasteride has also been evaluated in preliminary studies alongside finasteride and was found to perform significantly better than finasteride in improving female-pattern alopecia (Boersma et al. 2014). There is a paucity of data investigating the incidence of side effects relating to 5ARI use in women, however, it is important to note that women would not experience many of the side effects reported in male patients using 5ARIs, such as sexual dysfunction and gynecomastia, making these agents favorable options for treating hair loss in postmenopausal women. Doses are generally the same as with men: 1 mg finasteride orally or 0.5 mg dutasteride orally.

Conclusion

DHT blockers such as finasteride play a vital role in the clinical management of hair loss, particularly male-pattern baldness. By developing a deep understanding of the mechanisms of action, efficacy, and practical considerations associated with these treatments, practitioners can confidently integrate them into comprehensive hair loss management plans, tailoring their approach to the unique needs and goals of each patient. As the field of hair restoration continues to evolve, it is imperative for practitioners to stay abreast of emerging topical therapies and evidence-based practices. By continuously expanding their knowledge and skill set, practitioners can provide their patients with the most advanced and effective treatment options available. This commitment to ongoing learning and improvement is the hallmark of excellence in hair restoration, enabling practitioners to deliver the highest quality care to their patients and make a meaningful difference in their lives.

In the chapters that follow, we will delve deeper into the fascinating world of non-surgical hair restoration, exploring a range of innovative techniques and strategies that complement and enhance the efficacy of topical treatments. From the regenerative potential of platelet-rich plasma therapy to the stimulatory effects of low-level laser therapy and the synergistic benefits of microneedling, each modality offers unique opportunities to optimize hair growth and restore the confidence and well-being of patients. By embracing a comprehensive, multifaceted approach to hair restoration, we can unlock the full potential of non-surgical interventions and help patients achieve the healthy, vibrant hair they deserve.

Chapter 8

Platelet-Rich Plasma (PRP) Therapy

Bilal F. Hamzeh, Julyssa A. Renteria and Robert Dorfman

Introduction

Platelet-rich plasma (PRP) therapy has emerged as a promising non-surgical treatment for hair loss, harnessing the regenerative potential of the body's own growth factors to stimulate hair regrowth. This innovative approach involves the preparation and injection of a concentrated solution of platelets derived from the patient's own blood directly into the scalp. By delivering a potent blend of growth factors and bioactive molecules to the hair follicles, PRP therapy aims to enhance the hair growth cycle, improve follicular function, and promote the proliferation of specialized cells involved in hair production. This chapter provides an in-depth exploration of the mechanisms of action, preparation techniques, and clinical evidence supporting the use of PRP therapy in the management of hair loss. It also discusses patient selection, treatment protocols, and potential combinations with other hair restoration modalities, equipping practitioners with the knowledge and tools necessary to effectively incorporate PRP therapy into their clinical practice.

Mechanism of Action

The therapeutic potential of PRP in hair restoration lies in its ability to harness the regenerative properties of platelets and the growth factors they contain. Platelets, small, anucleate cells derived from megakaryocytes in the bone marrow, play a crucial role in the body's natural healing processes. When activated, platelets release a wide array of growth factors and bioactive molecules that orchestrate tissue repair, angiogenesis, and cellular proliferation. These growth factors, including platelet-derived growth factor (PDGF), transforming growth factor-beta (TGF-β), vascular endothelial growth factor (VEGF), and epidermal growth factor (EGF), have been implicated in the regulation of hair growth and the maintenance of hair follicle function (Garg and Manchanda 2017).

The precise mechanisms by which PRP promotes hair growth are not fully understood, but several key processes have been proposed. Firstly, the growth factors released by platelets are believed

DOI: 10.1201/9781032726397-8

to stimulate the proliferation and differentiation of dermal papilla cells, specialized mesenchymal cells located at the base of the hair follicle that play a pivotal role in regulating the hair growth cycle (Uebel et al. 2006). By enhancing the activity of dermal papilla cells, PRP may prolong the anagen (growth) phase of the hair cycle, leading to increased hair length and thickness. Secondly, PRP has been shown to promote angiogenesis, the formation of new blood vessels, via modulation of several biochemical pathways including the angiopoietin-1/Tie2 pathway (Mammoto et al. 2013). This increased vascularization improves the delivery of nutrients and oxygen to the hair follicles, creating a more favorable microenvironment for hair growth. Additionally, the growth factors in PRP may exert anti-inflammatory and anti-apoptotic effects on the hair follicles, protecting them from the deleterious impact of androgens and other factors that contribute to hair loss (Li et al. 2013).

Preparation and Administration

The preparation of PRP involves a multistep process designed to concentrate platelets from a sample of the patient's blood. The procedure begins with the collection of a small volume of blood, typically 20–60 mL, from the patient's peripheral vein. The blood is then placed in a specialized centrifugation device that separates the blood components based on their density. The first centrifugation step separates the red blood cells from the plasma and platelets, while the second centrifugation further concentrates the platelets, resulting in a platelet-rich plasma solution that contains 3–7 times the normal concentration of platelets found in whole blood (Dhurat and Sukesh 2014).

Once prepared, the PRP solution is carefully injected into the scalp using fine needles, targeting the affected areas of hair loss. The injections are typically performed under local anesthesia to minimize patient discomfort. The depth and distribution of the injections are critical factors in the success of the treatment, as the PRP must be delivered in close proximity to the hair follicles to exert its therapeutic effects. Practitioners may use various injection techniques, such as nappage (multiple superficial injections), papule (intradermal injections), or mesotherapy (a combination of superficial and intradermal injections), depending on the specific needs of the patient and the extent of hair loss (Alves and Grimalt 2018). Providers frequently recommend microneedling after PRP injection, in addition to peri-PRP microneedling, in order to introduce microlesions, initiating the coagulation cascade that activates platelets to release the growth factors of interest. Without the addition of post-PRP microneedling, it is thought that a considerable proportion of the benefit of PRP is left untapped. Without activation of the coagulation cascade initiated by microlesions introduced via microneedling, growth factors housed in platelet granules are not released. One study demonstrated the efficacy of microneedling using 1.5 mm long needles peri-PRP to achieve a clinically significant result (Yepuri and Venkataram 2021).

The optimal frequency and duration of PRP treatments for hair loss remain a subject of ongoing research. Most clinical protocols involve a series of three to six treatments, administered at monthly intervals, followed by maintenance treatments every 3–6 months to sustain the achieved results (Stevens and Khetarpal 2018). However, treatment plans may vary based on individual patient characteristics, the severity of hair loss, and the practitioner's clinical experience.

Clinical Evidence and Patient Outcomes

The efficacy of PRP therapy in the treatment of hair loss has been investigated in numerous clinical studies, yielding promising results. A systematic review and meta-analysis conducted by

Giordano et al. (2017) evaluated the outcomes of 12 studies involving a total of 295 patients with androgenetic alopecia treated with PRP. The analysis revealed a significant increase in hair density, hair thickness, and patient satisfaction following PRP treatment compared to baseline measurements. The pooled mean difference in hair density was +17.90 hairs/cm^2, while the mean difference in hair thickness was +0.22 mm, indicating a clinically meaningful improvement in hair growth parameters.

Alves and Grimalt (2018) conducted a randomized, double-blind, placebo-controlled trial to assess the efficacy and safety of PRP in the treatment of androgenetic alopecia. The study included 25 patients who received four sessions of PRP or placebo injections at monthly intervals. At 6 months post-treatment, the PRP group demonstrated a significant increase in hair density and hair thickness compared to the placebo group. The mean change in hair density was +19.2 hairs/cm^2 in the PRP group, compared to +4.8 hairs/cm^2 in the placebo group. The study also reported high patient satisfaction and a favorable safety profile, with no major adverse events.

Similar findings were reported by Gentile et al. (2015), who conducted a randomized, placebo-controlled trial involving 23 patients with androgenetic alopecia. The patients received three sessions of PRP or placebo injections at 30-day intervals. At the end of the 3-month follow-up period, the PRP group showed a significant increase in hair density and hair thickness compared to the placebo group. The mean increase in hair density was +27.7 hairs/cm^2 in the PRP group, compared to +3.2 hairs/cm^2 in the placebo group. The study also demonstrated a significant improvement in patient-reported outcomes, including overall satisfaction and perception of hair growth.

While these studies provide encouraging evidence for the efficacy of PRP in the treatment of androgenetic alopecia, it is important to acknowledge the limitations of the current body of research. Many of the available studies have relatively small sample sizes, short follow-up periods, and varying treatment protocols, making it challenging to draw definitive conclusions about the long-term effectiveness of PRP therapy. Additionally, the optimal concentration of platelets, frequency of treatments, and patient selection criteria remain to be fully elucidated. Further large-scale, well-designed clinical trials are needed to establish the standardized protocols and long-term outcomes of PRP therapy in the management of hair loss.

PRP has demonstrated efficacy not only in treating androgenetic alopecia but also other forms of alopecia, including scarring/immune-mediated alopecias, alopecia areata, and other forms of hair loss. PRP has shown efficacy in scarring alopecias, the mechanism of which remains unclear but is thought to result from modulation of the patient's immune system in addition to preventing scar formation and remodeling fibrotic tissue in scarring alopecias (Alser and Goutos 2018). In addition to regulating the activity of cytokines and interleukins that mediate inflammatory and anti-inflammatory conditions in the scalp, PRP is also thought to possess an anti-apoptotic mechanism, which is believed to play a potential role in the scar remodeling effect that poses a benefit in treating scarring alopecias (Moussa et al. 2017). Moreover, PRP has shown promise in the treatment of non-scarring, immune-mediated alopecias such as alopecia areata, demonstrating efficacy for 31.7–76% of patients, with the main side effect of treatment being injection site pain (Roohaninasab et al. 2021).

Combining PRP with Other Treatments

PRP therapy can be used as a standalone treatment for hair loss or in combination with other hair restoration modalities to enhance treatment outcomes. The synergistic effects of PRP with other therapies, such as minoxidil, finasteride, and low-level laser therapy (LLLT), have been explored in several studies.

Alves and Grimalt (2018) investigated the efficacy of a combination treatment involving PRP and LLLT in the management of androgenetic alopecia. The study included 36 patients who received three sessions of PRP injections at 30-day intervals, followed by LLLT twice a week for 16 weeks. The combination treatment resulted in a significant increase in hair density, hair thickness, and patient satisfaction compared to baseline measurements. The mean increase in hair density was +30.5 hairs/cm^2, while the mean increase in hair thickness was +0.21 mm, suggesting a potential additive effect of PRP and LLLT.

The combination of PRP with topical minoxidil has also been studied. Elena and Irina (2022) studied the effects of minoxidil and PRP dual therapy compared with either minoxidil or PRP monotherapy on hair growth in 69 men experiencing androgenetic alopecia. While either topical minoxidil 5% or PRP monotherapy significantly improved hair growth relative to placebo, the combination therapy was shown to be superior. Dual therapy was shown to increase hair density by 32% and hair shaft diameter by 26% while reducing the proportion of vellus hairs by 30% and of telogen hairs by 39%, which were all statistically significant findings relative to the control arm. Furthermore, a comparison of PRP and topical minoxidil combination therapy found that combination therapy exhibited a significant improvement in several parameters of hair growth including hair root thickness, density, hair shaft diameter, decreases in telogen and vellus hairs, and improvement in the anagen-to-telogen ratio of hairs. Other studies have produced similar findings. Shah et al. (2017) found PRP and minoxidil combination therapy to supersede the benefit observed with topical minoxidil monotherapy, and Alves and Grimalt (2018) also showed that PRP combination with standard therapies (minoxidil or 5ARIs) yielded a more pronounced clinical than monotherapy.

PRP is also being combined with extracellular matrix (ECM) substances such as ACell MatriStem and BioD. This combination, relative to PRP alone, allows treatments to be longer lasting, providing hair follicles not only with growth factors delivered via PRP but also with extracellular matrix components necessary for the structural support needed by hair follicles. Extracellular matrix products such as BioD and ACell, or synthetic ECM substances such as polydioxanone, are injected in a combination directly at the hair follicles, frequently followed immediately by microneedling. Some practitioners, such as Dr. Bauman at the Bauman Medical Center in Boca Raton, Florida, have reported that PRP plus ECM yields hair growth results that last significantly longer, up to 2 years, when compared with PRP alone (Bauman Medical 2025). These findings suggest that combining PRP with other established hair restoration therapies may offer additive or synergistic effects, potentially enhancing treatment outcomes. However, further research is needed to determine the optimal combination protocols and to evaluate the long-term efficacy and safety of these combined approaches.

Safety and Precautions

PRP therapy is generally considered a safe and well-tolerated treatment for hair loss, with a low risk of adverse events. As the procedure uses the patient's own blood, there is minimal risk of allergic reactions or rejection. The most common side effects associated with PRP injections include temporary swelling, redness, and discomfort at the injection sites, which typically resolve within a few days (Stevens and Khetarpal 2018).

To minimize the risk of complications, practitioners should adhere to strict aseptic techniques during the preparation and administration of PRP. Single-use, sterile equipment and proper skin disinfection prior to injections are essential to prevent infection. Patients with active scalp infections, bleeding disorders, or those taking anticoagulant medications should be carefully evaluated before undergoing PRP therapy. Additionally, patients should be informed about the potential risks and benefits of the treatment, and informed consent should be obtained prior to the procedure.

Contraindications

Although well-tolerated and generally regarded as a safe treatment for hair loss, PRP treatment does have contraindications that are important for practitioners to consider when assessing the candidacy of a patient for treatment (Badran and Sand 2018).

Contraindications to PRP therapy overlap with contraindications to general phlebotomy and include:

- Coagulation disorders
- Platelet dysfunction and thrombocytopenia
- Anticoagulant therapy such as aspirin, clopidogrel, warfarin, heparin, and direct oral anticoagulants
- Local infection at the site of blood harvesting or PRP injection site
- Hemodynamic instability
- Hepatitis
- Patients prone to keloid scar formation

Potentially major contraindications to PRP therapy include cancers and infections due to the increased risk of malignancy spread/metastases and spread of infections. Although recent research has demonstrated a potential therapeutic use of PRP in treating tissue infections (W. Zhang et al. 2019), in addition to existing research demonstrating a role of PRP in preventing infection through an antimicrobial action (Li and Li 2013), active infection is still generally considered a contraindication to the initiation of PRP therapy. The contraindication in cancer patients also holds; there is a paucity of research investigating the potential effect of PRP in cancer, and, as such, practitioners should generally consider active cancer to be a contraindication to the initiation of PRP therapy.

Conclusion

Platelet-rich plasma therapy represents a promising non-surgical approach to the management of hair loss, leveraging the regenerative potential of autologous growth factors to stimulate hair regrowth. By harnessing the biological properties of platelets, PRP aims to enhance the hair growth cycle, improve follicular function, and promote the proliferation of specialized cells involved in hair production. While the current body of evidence supports the efficacy of PRP in the treatment of androgenetic alopecia, further research is needed to establish standardized protocols, determine long-term outcomes, and explore the synergistic effects of combining PRP with other hair restoration modalities.

As the field of regenerative medicine continues to evolve, PRP therapy is poised to play an increasingly important role in the comprehensive management of hair loss. By staying abreast of the latest research and techniques, practitioners can effectively integrate PRP into their clinical practice, offering patients a safe, minimally invasive, and potentially transformative treatment option. As with any therapeutic intervention, a thorough understanding of the mechanisms of action, patient selection criteria, and treatment protocols is essential to optimize outcomes and ensure patient satisfaction.

In the following chapters, we will explore other innovative non-surgical approaches to hair restoration, including low-level laser therapy, microneedling, and nutritional interventions. By combining these modalities with PRP therapy and conventional treatments, practitioners can develop personalized, multifaceted treatment plans that address the unique needs of each patient, ultimately leading to more comprehensive and effective hair restoration outcomes.

Chapter 9

Laser Therapy

Bilal F. Hamzeh, Julyssa A. Renteria and Robert Dorfman

Introduction

Laser therapy, ranging from low-level laser therapy (LLLT) to advanced laser therapy, including, but not limited to, 1927 nm fractionated thulium laser treatment, has emerged as a promising option to induce hair growth in patients experiencing hair loss. LLLT is an innovative approach that harnesses the power of light to stimulate cellular processes and promote hair growth. By delivering low-level laser energy to the scalp, LLLT aims to enhance the hair growth cycle, improve follicular function, and increase hair density and thickness. Similarly, fractionated thulium, erbium, and CO_2 laser treatments, in addition to ultrasound-driven Alma TED, have emerged as non-invasive treatments for androgenetic alopecia. This chapter provides an overview of the known mechanisms of action, types of devices, and treatment protocols associated with LLLT; fractionated thulium, erbium, and CO_2 lasers; and ultrasound-based devices in the context of hair restoration. It also examines the clinical evidence supporting the efficacy of these treatment modalities and explores their potential as standalone treatments or in combination with other hair loss therapies. By understanding the principles and practical applications of laser therapies, practitioners can effectively incorporate this modality into their hair restoration treatment plans, offering patients a safe, non-invasive, and potentially effective option for managing hair loss.

LLLT Mechanism of Action

The therapeutic effects of LLLT in hair restoration, referred to as photobiomodulation, are believed to stem from its ability to modulate cellular processes and promote the proliferation and differentiation of hair follicle cells. The precise mechanisms by which LLLT stimulates hair growth are not fully understood, but several key processes have been proposed. LLLT covers a range of possible wavelengths, from red light through to infrared, and can induce biostimulation when applied at an appropriate energy level for a certain duration of time (Pillai and Mysore 2021). A biphasic dose–response has been described in relation to the clinical effects of LLLT, in which a subthreshold exposure has little clinical utility, an appropriate exposure induces biostimulation, and a suprathreshold exposure (in duration and/or light intensity) can paradoxically induce bio-inhibition. Although the application of light therapy for the treatment of hair loss is an emerging

DOI: 10.1201/9781032726397-9

and not yet fully understood field, it is hypothesized that this biphasic response to LLLT is related to the duality of effects of reactive oxygen species (ROS) and nitric oxide, which can both have stimulatory or inhibitory effects on tissues depending on the dose (Day and Suzuki 2006; Huang and Zheng 2006).

At the cellular level, LLLT is thought to enhance the function of mitochondria, the powerhouses of the cell, by increasing adenosine triphosphate (ATP) production (Chung et al. 2012). ATP is the primary energy currency of the cell, and its increased availability may support the metabolic demands of hair follicle cells during the growth phase. Additionally, LLLT has been shown to upregulate the expression of anti-inflammatory cytokines such as tissue growth factor-beta 1 and interleukin-10 and downregulate prostaglandins and other pro-inflammatory signaling molecules, potentially contributing to enhanced hair growth (Jimenez et al. 2014).

LLLT may also exert anti-inflammatory effects on the scalp, reducing the impact of inflammation-related hair loss. Inflammation has been implicated in the pathogenesis of androgenetic alopecia and other hair loss disorders, and the modulation of inflammatory pathways by LLLT may contribute to its therapeutic benefits (Avci et al. 2014).

Furthermore, LLLT has been proposed to stimulate the release of nitric oxide (NO) from cells, leading to vasodilation and increased blood flow to the scalp (Hamblin 2017). This enhanced microcirculation may improve the delivery of nutrients and oxygen to the hair follicles, creating a more favorable environment for hair growth.

Types of LLLT Devices

LLLT devices for hair restoration come in various forms, each with its advantages and considerations. The most common types of LLLT devices include:

- *Laser combs and brushes*: These handheld devices are designed to be combed or brushed through the hair, delivering low-level laser energy directly to the scalp. They offer the convenience of at-home use and allow for targeted treatment of specific areas of hair loss. However, the efficacy of laser combs and brushes may be limited by the relatively short contact time with the scalp and the need for consistent, manual application.
- *Laser caps and helmets*: These wearable devices provide a more hands-free approach to LLLT, allowing for longer treatment sessions and more comprehensive scalp coverage. Laser caps and helmets typically contain multiple laser diodes arranged to deliver energy evenly across the scalp. They offer the advantage of convenience and the ability to perform other tasks during treatment sessions. However, the cost of these devices may be higher than handheld options.
- *In-office laser systems*: Professional-grade laser systems are available for in-office use by trained practitioners. These devices often have higher power outputs and more advanced features compared to home-use devices. In-office LLLT treatments allow for personalized treatment plans, precise energy delivery, and the ability to combine LLLT with other hair restoration therapies. However, they require regular visits to the practitioner's office and may be associated with higher treatment costs.

When selecting a laser device, practitioners should consider factors such as the wavelength and power output of the laser, the size and coverage of the treatment area, and the ease of use for patients. It is essential to choose devices that have been specifically designed and tested for hair restoration purposes and have received appropriate regulatory clearances.

Treatment Protocols and Efficacy

The optimal treatment protocols for LLLT in hair restoration vary depending on the specific device used, the extent and type of hair loss, and individual patient characteristics (Lueangarun et al. 2021). However, some general guidelines have been established based on clinical studies and expert recommendations.

Most LLLT protocols involve regular treatment sessions, typically performed two to three times per week, for a minimum of 16–26 weeks (Jimenez et al. 2014). The duration of each session may range from a few minutes to 30 minutes or more, depending on the device and the size of the treatment area. Patients should be advised to follow the manufacturer's instructions carefully and to adhere to the recommended treatment schedule for optimal results.

The efficacy of LLLT in the treatment of hair loss has been investigated in numerous clinical studies, with promising results. A systematic review and meta-analysis conducted by Zarei et al. (2019) evaluated the outcomes of 21 studies including 12 evaluating LLLT. Multiple studies showed a significant increase in hair density and hair thickness, as well as patient-reported satisfaction with improvement of hair condition, following LLLT treatment compared to sham or placebo controls when controlling for parameters such as age and sex.

In a randomized, sham-controlled trial, Kim et al. (2013) investigated the efficacy of a helmet-type LLLT device in the treatment of androgenetic alopecia. The study included 40 patients who received LLLT or sham treatment twice weekly for 24 weeks. At the end of the treatment period, the LLLT group demonstrated a significantly greater increase in hair density compared to the sham group. The mean increase in hair density was +17.2 hairs/cm^2 in the LLLT group, compared to +2.1 hairs/cm^2 in the sham group.

Jimenez et al. (2014) conducted a randomized, double-blind, sham-controlled trial to evaluate the efficacy of a laser comb device in the treatment of male and female-pattern hair loss. The study included 128 patients who were treated with the laser comb or a sham device three times per week for 26 weeks. At the end of the treatment period, the laser comb group showed a significantly greater increase in terminal hair density compared to the sham group. The mean increase in terminal hair density was +19.3 hairs/cm^2 in the laser comb group, compared to +7.6 hairs/cm^2 in the sham group.

While these studies provide encouraging evidence for the efficacy of LLLT in the treatment of hair loss, it is important to acknowledge the limitations of the current body of research. Many of the available studies have relatively small sample sizes, short follow-up periods, and varying treatment protocols, making it challenging to draw definitive conclusions about the long-term effectiveness of LLLT. Additionally, the optimal wavelengths, power densities, and treatment durations for different types of hair loss remain to be fully elucidated. Further large-scale, well-designed clinical trials are needed to establish standardized protocols and long-term outcomes of LLLT in the management of hair loss.

Combination Therapies

LLLT can be used as a standalone treatment for hair loss or in combination with other hair restoration therapies to enhance treatment outcomes. The synergistic effects of LLLT with medications, such as minoxidil and finasteride, and with other non-invasive treatments, like PRP therapy, have been explored in several studies.

Ghanaat (2010) and Esmat et al. (2017) investigated the efficacy of a combination treatment involving LLLT and topical minoxidil in the management of androgenetic alopecia in female patients.

The study included 45 female patients who received LLLT through a helmet device and minoxidil 5% solution, minoxidil alone, or LLLT alone for four months. At the end of the treatment period, the combination group demonstrated a significantly greater improvement in hair density compared to the minoxidil-only or LLLT-only groups. While the number of follicles, assessed by ultrasound biomicroscopy, did not differ between the monotherapy groups, the combination group showed significantly higher hair density at two months ($p = 0.025$) and four months ($p < 0.001$).

As discussed in the previous chapter, Alves and Grimalt (2018) investigated the efficacy of a combination treatment involving LLLT and PRP in the management of androgenetic alopecia. The study included 36 patients who received three sessions of PRP injections at 30-day intervals, followed by LLLT twice a week for 16 weeks. The combination treatment resulted in a significant increase in hair density, hair thickness, and patient satisfaction compared to baseline measurements. The mean increase in hair density was +30.5 hairs/cm^2, while the mean increase in hair thickness was +0.21 mm, suggesting a potential additive effect of LLLT and PRP.

These findings suggest that combining LLLT with other established hair restoration therapies may offer additive or synergistic effects, potentially enhancing treatment outcomes. However, further research is needed to determine the optimal combination protocols and to evaluate the long-term efficacy and safety of these combined approaches.

Safety and Precautions

LLLT is generally considered a safe and well-tolerated treatment for hair loss, with a low risk of adverse events. The most common side effects associated with LLLT are mild and transient, including scalp irritation, redness, and itching (Avci et al. 2014). These side effects typically resolve spontaneously within a few days of treatment.

To minimize the risk of complications, practitioners should ensure that patients are properly instructed on the use of LLLT devices and adhere to the recommended treatment protocols. Patients should be advised to avoid looking directly into the laser light and to protect their eyes during treatment sessions. Individuals with a history of photosensitivity or those taking photosensitizing medications should be carefully evaluated before undergoing LLLT.

It is important to note that while LLLT is generally safe, it may not be suitable for all patients. Individuals with active scalp infections, cancerous lesions, or those undergoing chemotherapy or radiation therapy should not receive LLLT unless cleared by their treating physician. Pregnant women and individuals with epilepsy should also exercise caution and consult with their healthcare provider before starting LLLT.

1927 nm Fractionated Thulium Laser

The 1927 nm thulium laser is an emerging tool in the management of hair loss, offering an off-label yet novel approach in dermatology. Its use is based on its ability to target specific skin layers, promoting follicular regeneration and improving hair density. The non-ablative fractionated thulium laser induces targeted and controlled thermal damage that upregulates neocollagenesis and neovascularization, as with other laser treatment modalities. This wavelength is particularly adept at penetrating the skin to depths that affect the hair follicle environment, producing "microchannels in the skin, which increase topical growth factor and serum permeability to further induce hair growth and conversion from the telogen phase to the anagen phase." When applied to the scalp, the laser promotes controlled thermal injury that triggers a cascade of wound-healing processes. This includes the activation of stem cells within the hair follicles and the upregulation of growth factors such as VEGF and IGF-1, both of which are crucial for hair regeneration (Figure 9.1).

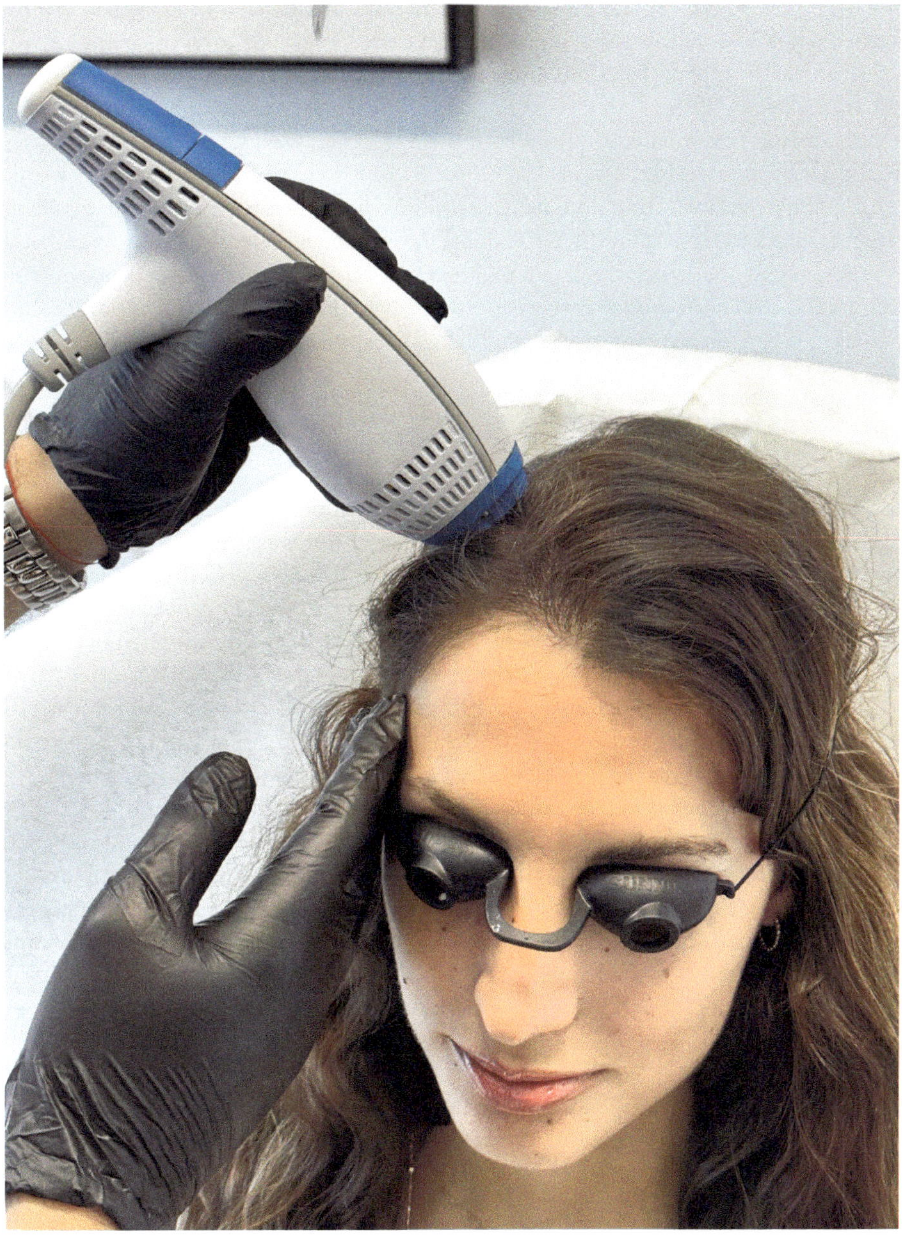

Figure 9.1 **1927 nm fractionated thulium laser.**

In my practice, I utilize a topical growth factor solution post-session to further enhance patient outcomes. As observed by Cho et al. (2018), patients who received topical application of a growth factor solution post-therapy experienced an increase in both hair density and thickness compared with patients who just received fractionated thulium laser therapy without post-session topical growth factor treatment, and also found increases in hair shaft density and diameter with thulium laser monotherapy (Cho et al. 2018). Similarly, it was also found that thulium laser, intrafollicular PDRN, and topical application of a growth factor solution were superior to mesotherapy with intrafollicular PDRN and topical growth factor solution alone (Cho et al. 2016). An overview of different factors and vitamins having differential effects on hair growth, many of which are included in topically applied solutions used in combination with laser therapies, is included in Table 9.1 (Dabek et al. 2019).

The frequency of fractionated thulium laser therapy varies, with Cho et al. (2018) demonstrating the efficacy of once-weekly sessions for 12 weeks. In my current practice, I use a frequency of one session per month (including non-ablative thulium laser therapy and topical application of a growth factor solution) for at least three sessions. Depending on patient preferences and outcomes, they can subsequently be transitioned to a maintenance phase in which the cadence of treatments decreases. As this treatment modality remains novel with exploration still underway, I recommend practitioners and patients explore varying regimens incorporating emerging laser therapies.

Fractionated Non-Ablative Erbium Glass Laser

The non-ablative erbium (Er) glass laser is another laser treatment modality that has demonstrated promise in the management of alopecia. Utilizing a 1550 nm wavelength and inducing thermal injury without tissue damage at an approximate depth of 0.4–2.0 mm, the non-ablative Er glass laser was shown to have a transient but beneficial effect on the anagen conversion of hair and the upregulation of WNT5A and beta-catenin in human subjects when administered over five sessions at 2-week intervals using 5 mJ (Kim et al. 2011). An additional study conducted by Bertin et al. (2018) assessed the combination of non-ablative Er glass laser application (8 sessions, 7 mJ) followed by topical finasteride (0.05%) and growth factor solution (bFGF, IGF-1, VEGF, Cu-peptides), and found improvement in hair regrowth and density via photomicrograph in all four patients.

Mechanistically, the non-ablative fractionated Er glass laser is thought to improve hair growth via cascades related, but not limited to upregulation, of Wnt/β-catenin and IGF pathways. Meephansan et al. assessed the effects of the 1550 nm Er glass laser on hair growth and signaling pathways in 23 patients. Histological and mRNA level assessment pre- and post-therapy involving 12 sessions of laser monotherapy at 2-week intervals yielded increases in the follicular unit, anagen phase hair count, and the anagen-to-telogen ratio but no upregulation of WNT10A or beta-catenin mRNA, suggesting alternative transcriptional mechanisms may be at play (Meephansan et al. 2018).

A similar study assessed the efficacy of 1540 nm non-ablative Er glass laser monotherapy in improving objective and subjective outcomes in the treatment of AGA in 51 patients and found that administration of 10 sessions at 2-week intervals yielded significant improvements in hair density and shaft thickness in the 47 patients who completed the trial (Alhattab et al. 2020). Lee et al. also found significant improvements using the 1550 nm Er laser in treating FPHL, showing marked increases in hair density (100 ± 14 to 157 ± 28 hairs cm^2, $P < 0.001$) and hair thickness (58 ± 12 μm to 75 ± 13 μm, $P < 0.001$), with a low incidence of adverse effects among the 27 participants, limited only to pruritus in two patients (7.4%) which resolved within 2 hours (Lee et al. 2011).

Table 9.1 Factors with Positive and Negative Effects on Hair Growth and Cycling

Category	*Positive Effects*	*Negative Effects*
Hormones	T3	Androgens/estrogens
Vitamins	Vitamin D3	
Growth factors	FGF-7	FGF-5
	IGF-1	FGF-18
	VEGF	TGF-β1
	PDGF	EGF
	HGF/SF	BMP2/4
	Thymosin β4	DKK1
	TGF-β2	BDNF
	Follistatin	
Cytokines		IL-1α
		IL-6
		IFN-γ
Others	Wnt	SP
	Arginine	CGRP
	Glucose	Exocannabinoids
	Glutamine	Endocannabinoids
	Spermidine	Histone H2A
	Carnitine tartrate	Histone H4
	Cyclosporine A	

Source: Adapted from RJ Dabek et al., Laser-assisted hair regrowth: Fractional laser modalities for the treatment of androgenic alopecia, *Plast Reconstr Surg Glob Open.* 2019;7(4):e2157, with permission.

Abbreviations: BMP, bone morphogenetic protein; BDNF, brain-derived neurotrophic factor; CGRP, calcitonin gene-related peptide; DKK1, Dickkopf-related protein 1; EGF, epidermal growth factor; FGF, fibroblast growth factor; HGF/SF, hepatocyte growth factor/scatter factor; IFN -γ, interferon gamma; IGF-1, insulin-like growth factor; IL, interleukin; PDGF, platelet-derived growth factor; SP, substance P; T3, triiodothyronine; TGF, transforming growth factor; VEGF, vascular endothelial growth factor.

Although still an emerging treatment modality, the fractionated non-ablative Er glass laser has demonstrated promise in the treatment of male and female-pattern hair loss both as a monotherapy and in combination with pharmacotherapeutics and growth factor solutions. Limitations exist with respect to understanding the underlying mechanism of action, as is generally the case with light therapies for hair loss, but the low incidence of adverse effects, non-invasive nature, and tolerability make the non-ablative Er glass laser a valuable tool and a treatment modality that practitioners and patients can explore.

Fractionated CO_2 Laser

Fractionated CO_2 lasers operate by emitting laser beams that create microscopic thermal zones (MTZs) of controlled damage surrounded by unaffected tissue. This pattern facilitates rapid healing and minimizes downtime compared to fully ablative lasers. The primary wavelength for CO_2 lasers is approximately 10,600 nm, which is highly absorbed by water in the skin, leading to precise ablation and thermal remodeling of the dermal layers. Mechanistically, fractionated laser therapies such as CO_2 laser therapy induce microscopic injuries that cultivate an inflammatory perifollicular environment that promotes hair growth. Disruption of skin layers also promotes enhanced delivery of topical drugs (Dabek et al. 2019).

Shen et al. (2023) conducted a meta-analysis demonstrating the efficacy of non-ablative fractionated CO_2 lasers in improving hair growth in patients with alopecia areata being treated with topical minoxidil or cortisol. Fractionated laser therapy was also effective in treating alopecia areata alone (RR 10.33, 95% CI 2.07–51.36, $p = 0.004$), and had improved outcomes relative to either topical minoxidil or topical corticosteroid monotherapies. Moreover, a study conducted by Salah et al. (2019) investigated the effect of combined ablative fractionated CO2 laser with and without topical minoxidil for male androgenetic alopecia and found that hair thickness of both thin and thick hair increased in the combination group relative to the minoxidil group.

Alma TED™

Alma TED™ is a novel therapeutic approach to hair loss that utilizes low-frequency ultrasound, pressure, and electrostimulation to stimulate hair follicles and induce growth, with excellent tolerability and an absence of side effects often noted with more established treatment options such as minoxidil and finasteride. Ultrasound has been explored as an option to increase the efficacy of topically applied medications in the past, and Alma TED represents its recent application to the field of hair growth (Seah and Teo 2018). As this is a novel treatment modality, there is a scarcity of peer-reviewed studies assessing the efficacy of Alma TED relative to pharmacotherapies and targeted laser therapies. The mechanism of Alma TED is similar to that of other non-ablative therapies: it stimulates hair follicles and has an additional benefit of increasing the permeability of the epidermal layer, enhancing the delivery of growth factors and sera applied topically (termed transepidermal delivery, or TED).

One study evaluating the efficacy of Alma TED in 50 participants with hair loss ranging in severity and etiology, including MPHL/FPHL, telogen effluvium, autoimmune, lichen planopilaris, and central centrifugal scarring hair loss, identified a 98% positive response rate and an 89% improvement in hair density. Patients with active infections around the treatment area or known malignancy were excluded. Patients were treated for a total of three sessions, each structured as follows:

Step 1: Priming with Alma TED (2 minutes)
Step 2: Topical application of the peptide-based Hair Care Formula
Step 3: Treating with Alma TED (2 minutes)

The study found no adverse reactions or complications associated with the treatment, and was distinguished in the favorable response observed in patients experiencing scarring alopecias, reducing shedding and improving subjective and objective parameters of hair density as soon as 30 days after termination of treatment (Dy 2023).

A similar study was conducted in a cohort of eleven patients, eight women and three men, following a similar protocol. While results were favorable, with 100% of participants reporting decreased shedding and increased growth following treatment, objective measures show a potential limitation in the durability of results. The terminal:vellus ratio across the entirety of the scalp was shown to increase by 48% on the day 30 follow-up assessment relative to baseline, but subsequently reduced to an improvement of 11% relative to baseline at 90 days (Desai 2023). Further evaluation is needed to better characterize the limitations of Alma TED and potential adjunctive treatments that can be used in tandem to help improve the longevity of results observed with this treatment modality.

As an FDA-cleared treatment, Alma TED is a potential tool that can be utilized by practitioners, in tandem with other therapy modalities and adjunctively with topical growth sera to bolster the hair growth potential of patients. Alma TED, being a non-invasive and low commitment form of therapy for patients, requiring short sessions that can be administered in a single visit, is an avenue that should be explored by practitioners and discussed with patients. As with all treatment modalities, providers and patients should work together to assess treatment options, risks, and desired outcomes while assessing which treatment options they should explore. As previously mentioned, further research is necessary to better delineate the optimal use cases and treatment regimens involving Alma TED to best leverage its potential in clinical settings, affording patients the best possible outcomes.

Indications and Contraindications

Laser therapy is generally indicated as a safe and efficacious treatment modality for many forms of alopecia in addition to other dermatological conditions. Beyond the demonstrated efficacy of laser therapy in the treatment of androgenetic alopecia alongside other treatment modalities, laser therapy has also shown utility in the management of other forms of alopecia including alopecia areata (Jean-Pierre et al. 2024). The 308 nm excimer laser, for example, is a therapy that boasts an immunosuppressive effect that is thought to result in T cell apoptosis. This effect is beneficial in the management of alopecia areata due to the auto-immune etiology of this form of alopecia. One study conducted in 2007 demonstrated the efficacy of the 308 nm excimer laser; of the patients recruited to the study, all those with alopecia areata experienced hair growth (Zakaria et al. 2004). There is a paucity of data demonstrating the efficacy of light therapy in the treatment of other forms of alopecia, such as scarring alopecia, and further research is necessary to elucidate the potential benefits.

In terms of contraindications, laser and ultrasound therapies are generally well tolerated and there are few contraindications to their use, most of them depending on practitioner judgment on a case-by-case basis.

Some potential contraindications to the use of laser therapies for alopecia include:

- Medications that cause photosensitization, including tetracyclines such as doxycycline, nitrofurantoin, retinoids, and amiodarone. Some of these medications, such as doxycycline and retinoids, are widely used in dermatology and do not often lead to photosensitization that would prevent the use of laser therapies (Kerstein et al. 2014). Determination of patient candidacy must be done clinically on a case-by-case basis, dependent on symptoms of photosensitivity if present.

- Histologically demonstrated carcinoma.
- Epilepsy.
- Active infection.
- History of cancer in the region to be treated.
- Pregnancy.

These are not absolute contraindications, as there are very few, if any absolute contraindications to the use of laser therapy on the scalp to treat alopecia, although there are contraindications with respect to applying laser therapies elsewhere on the body (Navratil and Kymplova 2002). As with many treatments of alopecia, practitioner judgment is ultimately required in cases of potential contraindications to any therapy modality for non-surgical hair restoration.

Conclusion

Laser therapy represents a promising non-invasive approach to the management of hair loss, harnessing the power of light to stimulate cellular processes and promote hair growth. By modulating inflammation, enhancing microcirculation, and stimulating the release of growth factors, laser therapy aims to enhance the hair growth cycle and improve follicular function. Moreover, the use of light and ultrasound therapies in the clinical management of hair loss not only show promise as monotherapies, but also as combination therapies and as mechanisms through which to improve transdermal drug delivery, all of which may have a compounding beneficial effect in the treatment of alopecia.

While the current body of evidence supports the efficacy of LLLT in the treatment of androgenetic alopecia and other forms of hair loss, further research is needed to establish standardized protocols, determine long-term outcomes, and explore the synergistic effects of combining LLLT with other hair restoration modalities. Other modalities of laser therapies, such as carbon dioxide, erbium, and 1927 nm thulium laser, as well as the novel Alma TED ultrasound-based treatment, represent emerging treatment options either alone or adjunctively with other treatment modalities.

As the field of hair restoration continues to evolve, LLLT and other light therapies are poised to play an increasingly important role in the comprehensive management of hair loss. By staying abreast of the latest research and technological advancements, practitioners can effectively integrate laser therapies into their clinical practice, offering patients a safe, non-invasive, and potentially transformative treatment option. As with any therapeutic intervention, a thorough understanding of the mechanisms of action, patient selection criteria, and treatment protocols is essential to optimize outcomes and ensure patient satisfaction.

In the following chapters, we will delve into other innovative non-surgical approaches to hair restoration, including microneedling and nutritional interventions. By combining these modalities with laser therapies, conventional treatments, and emerging therapies, practitioners can develop personalized, multifaceted treatment plans that address the unique needs of each patient, ultimately leading to more comprehensive and effective hair restoration outcomes.

Chapter 10

Nutritional and Supplemental Therapy

Bilal F. Hamzeh, Haley Guinan, Julyssa A. Renteria, Robert Dorfman and Sophia Kurian

Introduction

Nutritional and supplemental therapies play a crucial role in the comprehensive management of hair loss, serving as complementary approaches to support the efficacy of other non-surgical hair restoration treatments. By addressing nutritional deficiencies, promoting healthy hair growth, and minimizing the impact of factors that contribute to hair loss, these therapies offer a holistic approach to hair restoration. This chapter explores the role of vitamins, minerals, and other essential nutrients in maintaining healthy hair, as well as the evidence supporting the use of specific supplements in the treatment of hair loss. It also discusses dietary modifications and lifestyle interventions that can optimize hair health and enhance the outcomes of non-surgical hair restoration treatments. By incorporating nutritional and supplemental therapies into their treatment plans, practitioners can provide patients with a well-rounded approach to managing hair loss and achieving optimal results.

Role of Vitamins and Minerals

Vitamins and minerals play essential roles in the growth and maintenance of healthy hair. Deficiencies in certain nutrients can contribute to hair loss and impair the efficacy of hair restoration treatments. Therefore, it is crucial for practitioners to assess patients' nutritional status and address any deficiencies as part of a comprehensive hair loss management plan.

1. *Vitamin D*: Vitamin D is a fat-soluble vitamin that plays a crucial role in hair follicle cycling and differentiation. Low levels of vitamin D have been associated with various forms of hair loss, including androgenetic alopecia (AGA) and telogen effluvium (Gerkowicz et al. 2017). Vitamin D supplementation has been shown to promote hair growth and improve the outcomes of other hair restoration therapies (Sattar et al. 2021).

DOI: 10.1201/9781032726397-10

2. *Biotin (vitamin B7)*: Biotin is a water-soluble B vitamin that is essential for the metabolism of fatty acids and the production of keratin, the primary protein component of hair. Biotin deficiency can lead to hair loss, and supplementation has been shown to improve hair thickness and overall hair health (Patel et al. 2017).
3. *Iron*: Iron is a mineral that plays a crucial role in the synthesis of hemoglobin, which carries oxygen to the hair follicles. Iron deficiency anemia has been associated with telogen effluvium and diffuse hair loss (Park et al. 2013). Correcting iron deficiency through dietary modifications and supplementation can help restore hair growth and improve the outcomes of hair restoration treatments.
4. *Zinc*: Zinc is a trace mineral that is involved in numerous biological processes, including hair follicle development and keratinization. Zinc deficiency can lead to hair loss and impaired wound healing (Gupta et al. 2014). Zinc supplementation has been shown to improve hair growth in patients with androgenetic alopecia and other forms of hair loss (Karashima et al. 2012).

Other important nutrients for hair health include vitamin A, vitamin C, vitamin E, selenium, and essential fatty acids. A balanced diet rich in fruits, vegetables, lean proteins, and healthy fats can help to ensure an adequate intake of these nutrients and support optimal hair growth.

Recommended Supplements

In addition to addressing nutrient deficiencies, certain supplements have been specifically studied for their potential benefits in the treatment of hair loss. These supplements may be recommended by practitioners as part of a comprehensive hair restoration plan.

1. *Marine protein supplements*: Marine proteins, such as those derived from fish or shellfish, are rich in essential amino acids, minerals, and omega-3 fatty acids. These nutrients are crucial for hair follicle function and the production of keratin. A randomized, double-blind, placebo-controlled study by Ablon and Kogan (2016) found that a marine protein supplement containing a blend of shark cartilage, oyster extract, and fish oil significantly improved hair growth and hair thickness in patients with thinning hair.
2. *Saw palmetto*: Saw palmetto (*Serenoa repens*) is a plant extract that has been widely studied for its potential benefits in the treatment of androgenetic alopecia. Saw palmetto is believed to work by inhibiting the activity of 5-alpha reductase, the enzyme responsible for converting testosterone to dihydrotestosterone (DHT), a key factor in the development of male-pattern baldness (Evron et al. 2020). A meta-analysis by Murugusundram (2009) concluded that saw palmetto supplementation could improve hair count and hair density in patients with androgenetic alopecia.
3. *Pumpkin seed oil*: Pumpkin seed oil is rich in phytosterols, which are plant-based compounds that have been shown to inhibit 5-alpha reductase activity and reduce DHT levels in the scalp (Ibrahim 2021). A randomized, placebo-controlled, double-blind study by Cho et al. (2014) found that oral supplementation with pumpkin seed oil for 24 weeks significantly increased hair count and hair thickness in men with androgenetic alopecia.
4. *Green tea extract:* Green tea extract is rich in polyphenols, particularly epigallocatechin-3-gallate (EGCG), which has been shown to have anti-inflammatory and antioxidant properties (Akbarnejad 2023). These properties may help to protect hair follicles from damage and promote hair growth. A study by Esfandiari and Kelly (2005) found that a combination of green tea extract and topical minoxidil was more effective in treating androgenetic alopecia than minoxidil alone.

When recommending supplements, practitioners should consider the quality, purity, and safety of the products, as well as potential interactions with medications and other supplements (Drake et al. 2023). It is essential to educate patients on the proper dosage and administration of supplements and to monitor for any adverse reactions.

The challenge with alternative treatments is that the supplement industry is largely unregulated, particularly in the United States, meaning it is very difficult to assess the precise dosage and purity of unregulated over-the-counter agents, particularly herbal supplements, not regulated by the FDA (Starr 2015). Moreover, many instances of adverse reactions to herbal supplements are reported in the literature, such as hepatotoxicity. For example, the predominant catechin in green tea, EGCG, is associated with cases of hepatotoxicity (Acosta et al. 2023). In fact, herbal and dietary supplements account for 20% of cases of clinically apparent liver injury in the United States (Navarro et al. 2017). With the paucity of evidence relating to the safety of purified and high-dose phytochemical extracts, in addition to the lack of randomized controlled trials, FDA regulation, and third-party testing, great care should be taken when patients initiate adjunctive therapy with over-the-counter herbal supplements.

Topical Alternative Treatments

As with pharmacotherapies indicated to treat hair loss, herbal and alternative treatments for hair loss are often used topically in addition to orally. Patients often attempt to address hair loss first through the use of oral and topical natural remedies before scheduling a consultation to address the issue with a practitioner. Moreover, alternative treatments can often continue to play a role in a patient's treatment regimen even after initiating formal pharmacotherapy, and, as such, practitioners should maintain familiarity with commonly used agents, their mechanisms of action, and potential benefits and uses.

Naturally occurring alternative medicines have a long history of use in treating hair loss and continue to play a significant role in modern solutions to hair loss. Alternative treatments are commonly used adjunctively with pharmacotherapies such as minoxidil and finasteride and can often be a first-line approach for patients seeking to treat alopecia before seeking medical treatment. Commonly used alternative treatments, including methods of use, mechanism of action, and efficacy, are described next.

1. *Rosemary oil*: *Rosmarinus officinalis*, or rosemary, is a plant native to the Mediterranean region. Historically, rosemary oil has been used both topically and orally to treat conditions ranging from headaches, neuralgia, and hair loss to insomnia, depression, and rheumatic disease (Ghasemzadeh and Hosseinzadeh 2020). The active constituents of rosemary oil are thought to improve tissue perfusion and boast anti-inflammatory, antimicrobial, and antioxidant benefits via the combined entourage effect of phytochemicals (Presley et al. 2021).
   - *Usage*: Rosemary oil is typically applied topically to the scalp. Often, oil extracted from *Rosmarinus officinalis* is diluted in a carrier oil and sold for topical administration. Rosemary oil marketed for the treatment of hair loss is also frequently sold in oils combined with other herbal extracts, vitamins, and fatty acids. Rosemary oil has also been used historically to treat myalgias, headaches, arthritis, and neuropathic pain, in addition to its use in gastrointestinal conditions such as constipation and indigestion.
   - *Mechanism of action*: Rosemary oil is known to contain several active constituents that have a collective beneficial effect on promoting hair growth. These compounds include carnosic and rosmarinic acids, which act as antioxidants, ursolic acid, which has been

found to inhibit 5-alpha reductase, and eucalyptol, promoting an antioxidant and vasodilatory action (Huang et al. 2019). The crude extract of rosemary has been shown to possess anti-inflammatory action by inhibiting leukocytes and exudation in addition to blocking inflammatory mediators such as interleukin 1-beta (IL-1β), myeloperoxidase (MPO), and tumor necrosis factor-alpha (TNF-alpha) (Benincá et al. 2011). Furthermore, rosemary extract has been shown to reduce platelet aggregation by 82%, nitric oxide by 71.8%, and free radical generation by 91.8% (Yimam et al. 2017). This anti-inflammatory effect produces favorable conditions in the treatment of androgenetic alopecia, which can involve perifollicular inflammatory infiltrate (Bin Rubaian et al. 2024).
   - *Clinical data*: A randomized comparative trial by Panahi et al. (2015) found rosemary oil to be as effective as 2% minoxidil in promoting hair growth in patients with AGA, but with a lower incidence of side effects such as scalp itching. Moreover, animal and cell culture models have shown some active constituents of rosemary oil, particularly 12-methoxy carnosic acid, as possessing 5-alpha reductase inhibitor activity, reversing hair loss induced by androgens in mice and preventing androgen-dependent growth of a cell line, LNCaP (Murata et al. 2013). Given the tolerability, history of human use, and positive benefits associated with the use of rosemary oil, it may serve as an important adjunct in the clinical management of hair loss and restoration.
2. *Peppermint oil*: *Mentha piperita*, or peppermint, is a plant native to Europe that has historically been used as a carminative to relieve flatulence and as a gastric stimulant. In fact, peppermint oil is still used today in over-the-counter preparations indicated for the treatment of irritable bowel syndrome (IBS). In the context of hair growth, peppermint oil is mostly used as a topical agent.
   - *Usage*: Peppermint oil is extracted from *Mentha piperita* and diluted in a carrier oil for topical administration. Peppermint oil is generally well tolerated and is not often associated with dermatological effects related to applications such as pruritus and irritation. Peppermint oil marketed for hair growth is often sold in formulations that combine it with other natural oils indicated to promote hair growth, such as castor oil and rosemary oil.
   - *Mechanism of action*: Menthol and eucalyptol are responsible for the vasodilatory effect of peppermint oil, while menthone and other bioactive constituents such as limonene are known to impart antioxidant and anti-inflammatory effects. Menthol is thought to induce vasodilation and increased perfusion at interrogated skin sites via a complex interplay of mediators including nitric oxide (NO), endothelium-derived hyperpolarization factors (EDHFs), and sensory nerve responses (Silva 2020). As with minoxidil and other vasodilatory compounds, this mechanism of action allows for increased perfusion of hair follicles, yielding an environment that favorably promotes hair growth via mechanisms that have not been very well defined.
   - *Clinical data*: While clinical data exploring the efficacy of topical peppermint oil in humans with AGA is limited, there are limited clinical data demonstrating the efficacy of topical menthol as a vasodilator (Craighead and Alexander 2016), in addition to data in animals that exhibit promise with respect to the potential use of peppermint oil in AGA (Panahi et al. 2015). One animal study conducted in mice found peppermint oil to yield greater hair growth than any other assessed compound, including a standardized formulation of jojoba oil and 3% topical minoxidil, with increased hair thickness and hair follicle number and depth, thought to be associated with the

significant elevations in alkaline phosphatase (ALP) and insulin-like growth factor-1 (IGF-1) activity associated with peppermint oil compared with jojoba oil and topical minoxidil (Oh et al. 2014).

3. *Pumpkin seed oil*: The seeds of *Cucurbita pepo*, or pumpkin, have a long history of use for medicinal purposes and are a valuable source of fatty acids including omega fatty acids, proteins, and vitamins such as carotenoids and tocopherols, in addition to trace elements such as zinc and selenium (Shaban et al. 2017). Pumpkin seed oil has also been shown to be beneficial in treating benign prostatic hyperplasia via the inhibition of androgens through phytosterols present in the oil, a benefit that has also been applied to the treatment of alopecia.
   - *Usage*: Pumpkin seed oil is a natural remedy rich in antioxidants and essential fatty acids, including β-carotene, lutein, γ- and β-tocopherols, linolenic acid, and phytosterols. It has been used historically in various countries to treat conditions like prostate disorders, hair loss, and cardiovascular issues. Typically, it is administered orally in capsule form or applied topically. Among other uses, pumpkin seed oil has been used to treat benign prostatic hyperplasia; two studies have demonstrated the efficacy of pumpkin seed oil administered to rats following exogenous testosterone-induced prostate hyperplasia (Gossell-Williams and O'Connor et al. 2006; Tsai et al. 2006). These antiandrogenic effects would pose the same benefit in treating hair loss; pharmacotherapeutics such as finasteride have similarly shown benefits in treating both prostate issues and hair loss, as both conditions are androgen-mediated.
   - *Mechanism of action*: The key active components, β-sitosterol and linolenic acid, inhibit 5-alpha reductase, an enzyme involved in the conversion of testosterone to DHT, which contributes to AGA. By reducing IL-6 activity, pumpkin seed oil helps prevent hair loss and promotes hair growth (Carbin et al. 1990). Pumpkin seed oil is also known to contain zinc, which acts as an antioxidant via neutralization of free radicals and by engaging iron and copper binding sites present on macromolecules (Amara et al. 2008), playing an important role in DNA stability and repair mechanisms crucial for hair growth. Additionally, tocopherol and other constituents present in pumpkin seed oil have been shown to rescue hemodynamic instability via a nitric oxide-dependent pathway (El-Mosallamy et al. 2012).
   - *Clinical data*: Studies have shown that pumpkin seed oil capsules were effective in increasing hair count and hair thickness in men with AGA after 24 weeks. Side effects are generally mild, such as abdominal discomfort or itching, but no significant changes in liver enzymes, creatinine, blood pressure, or testosterone levels were observed. One randomized controlled trial compared the efficacy of once-daily application of 1 mL pumpkin seed oil to the scalp to 5% minoxidil topical foam in treating female-pattern hair loss and found no significant difference, with both treatments showing a significant increase in hair shaft density and vellus hairs (Ibrahim et al. 2021). In men, pumpkin seed oil has been shown to significantly increase hair growth, yielding statistically significant improvements in self-reported satisfaction and in mean hair count (40%) when compared to placebo (Cho et al. 2014).
4. *Saw palmetto*: *Serenoa repens*, or saw palmetto, is a native palm tree that is native to the southeastern United States. Boasting DHT-inhibiting properties, saw palmetto has historically been used as a natural remedy for prostate hyperplasia and hair loss, much like other herbal supplements and pharmacotherapies with a principal action of reducing levels of circulating DHT. It has also historically been used to treat infertility and underdeveloped

breasts in women, as an appetite stimulant, a nerve sedative, and an expectorant, with many uses improving the health and function of the genitourinary system.

- *Usage*: Saw palmetto (*Serenoa repens*) is a plant extract traditionally used for conditions such as benign prostatic hyperplasia (BPH) and hair loss. It is available as an oral supplement or topical formulation. Although the use of saw palmetto has seen a decline in the United States, the herb is still widely used in Europe, particularly in Germany, where it is still considered by many to be a first-line treatment of BPH. Use in Germany is so widespread, in fact, that a standard has been set such that lipophilic extracts must contain 85–95% fatty acids and sterols, thought to be the principal active constituents in the herb. Saw palmetto is available as a prescription drug called Permixon, shown in clinical trials to be well tolerated and effective against BPH.
- *Mechanism of action*: The extract inhibits 5-alpha reductase, thereby reducing DHT levels and promoting hair growth. By lowering DHT, saw palmetto supports both prostate health and hair retention (Carbin et al. 1990; Anastassakis 2022). While 5-alpha reductase inhibitors such as finasteride and dutasteride exert a competitive inhibitory effect on one or both isoenzymes of 5-alpha reductase, saw palmetto has been shown to inhibit both forms of the enzyme in a noncompetitive manner (Raynaud et al. 2002). Other studies have demonstrated mixed action of the lipid and sterol constituents of the plant, demonstrating differential noncompetitive and uncompetitive inhibition of one or both isoenzymes of 5-alpha reductase in porcine tissues (Palin et al. 1998). Outside of the antiandrogenic effect of saw palmetto, lipid extracts of the plant have also been shown to inhibit binding of alpha-1 adrenergic receptors, a pharmacodynamic property that may pose additional benefits in the management of benign prostatic hyperplasia and urinary symptoms (Goepel et al. 1999). Vanilloids present in the plant also inhibit TRPV1 receptors, which may play a role in the pathogenesis of urinary diseases (Birder et al. 2001).
- *Clinical data*: Saw palmetto is widely used, with approximately 2.5 million US adults taking it regularly, but the clinical evidence supporting its use in hair growth is ambiguous (Roehrborn 2006). The largest randomized controlled trial to date evaluated the efficacy of oral saw palmetto extract against 1 mg oral finasteride and found that while 38% of patients showed improvement in hair growth with saw palmetto, this was inferior to the 68% that saw improvement with finasteride. This study also found that while finasteride was effective across the entirety of the scalp, saw palmetto showed the most benefits, most commonly at the vertex (Rossi et al. 2012). Both topical and oral forms of saw palmetto extract have been shown to be well tolerated and to boast antiandrogenic and antioxidant effects (Morganti et al. 1998). The use of a standardized saw palmetto extract, Lambdapil, also containing cysteine and biotin, was shown to have positive effects on patient satisfaction and hair growth assessed via phototrichogram in men experiencing AGA (Narda et al. 2017). Although some studies show potential, more robust trials are required to validate these claims.

5. *Caffeine extract*: Caffeine is frequently used in personal care commercial formulations with indications ranging from rejuvenation of skin to promotion of hair growth. With a long history of human use as a stimulant, caffeine has a well-established safety index in humans and has been explored to treat conditions ranging from headaches to narcolepsy. Caffeine present in nutritional supplements is often synthetic, but can be extracted from a variety of plants, including green tea and coffee most commonly. Caffeine use has also been associated with a decreased risk of dementia and cognitive decline, among other purported benefits.

- *Usage*: Caffeine is commonly found in coffee beans, the seeds of the *Coffea* plant, and is widely known for its stimulant properties. In hair care, caffeine extract is often applied topically in shampoos and sera to combat hair thinning and loss. Caffeine extracts are often present in shampoos, conditioners, and other personal care products purported to improve hair growth and density. Caffeine is capable of diffusing through the skin in humans and has almost complete oral bioavailability, making the administration of caffeine topically or orally feasible routes for targeting hair loss (Völker et al. 2020). Outside of its widespread use as a stimulant and the potential use for hair growth, caffeine has been used as a thermogenic and weight loss supplement, a cognitive enhancer, and to treat headaches, where it is frequently used in over-the-counter medications in combination with NSAIDs or aspirin.
- *Mechanism of action*: Caffeine enhances microvascular perfusion by upregulating cyclic adenosine monophosphate (cAMP), leading to better blood flow in the scalp and improved nutrient delivery to hair follicles. The mechanism through which caffeine upregulates cAMP is via inhibition of phosphodiesterases, which promotes metabolic activity and cellular proliferation (Chen et al. 2024). In a hair organ culture model, caffeine was shown to stimulate hair growth and upregulate the proliferation of keratinocytes, counteracting testosterone-induced expression of TGF-beta in a tissue model of male androgenetic alopecia (Philpott et al. 1994).
- *Clinical data*: Although caffeine's systemic effects are well studied, data supporting its use in hair loss treatments is still emerging. Early studies show it can help stimulate hair growth in certain cases, but excessive consumption (more than 400 mg/day) can lead to side effects such as fatigue, irritability, and nervousness. Outside of organ culture models, there is clinical data demonstrating the utility of caffeine in treating AGA. One such study compared the topical application of a 0.2% caffeine serum to 5% minoxidil and showed a mean improvement in the anagen ratio via trichogram of 10.59% in the caffeine group compared with 11.68% in the minoxidil group, both demonstrating significant improvements that did not show a statistical difference, demonstrating the noninferiority of caffeine compared with minoxidil in improving this metric (Dhurat et al. 2017). An additional in vitro study that cultivated follicles from biopsies taken from the vertices of 14 men experiencing AGA showed that caffeine applied at concentrations of 0.001% and 0.005% rescued testosterone-induced suppression of follicle growth (Fischer et al. 2007). Still, there is certainly a paucity of clinical data demonstrating the efficacy of caffeine in the treatment of AGA and further research is required.

6. *Melatonin*: Melatonin is an endogenous neurohormone secreted by the pineal gland, skin, lymphocytes, and gastrointestinal tract that plays a role in the regulation of the circadian rhythm and hormone regulation in addition to having antioxidant properties. It is frequently used in over-the-counter formulations indicated to promote sleep and treat insomnia, and is available as a prescription drug across the world indicated to treat insomnia and circadian dysregulation. The synthetic melatonin analog ramelteon, selectively agonizing MT1 and MT2 receptors, was marketed under the trade name Rozerem for the treatment of insomnia. More recently, melatonin has been investigated for indications beyond insomnia, where it has demonstrated some potential promise as a possible treatment for hair loss.
   - *Usage*: Melatonin is a hormone primarily known for its role in regulating sleep cycles. In addition to its systemic effects, melatonin is also applied topically to reduce oxidative stress in both the skin and hair. This application has gained attention for its potential in treating hair loss conditions like AGA. One systematic review found evidence

that topical administration of melatonin, unlike oral administration indicated for the treatment of insomnia, had a positive effect on scalp hair growth, hair density, and hair thickness. There is also some evidence that both topical formulations of melatonin, used as a spray at concentrations ranging from 0.0033% to 0.1%, and oral forms, consumed orally at a dose of 1.5 mg twice daily, may have some benefit in treating androgenetic alopecia in men (Babadjouni et al. 2023). The potential side effect of somnolence, however, may make oral dosing of melatonin for alopecia difficult and treatment-limiting.

- *Mechanism of action*: Melatonin acts as a powerful antioxidant, protecting hair follicles from oxidative damage and photodamage, which may help slow the progression of AGA. In addition to this, melatonin is synthesized within the hair follicles, especially during the anagen phase, where it may play a role in hair-cycle regulation. Research has identified the presence of MT2 receptors and nuclear RORα receptors in hair follicles, which suggests that melatonin helps modulate hair growth through these pathways. Melatonin further promotes DNA repair and reduces apoptosis, potentially serving as a self-cytoprotective mechanism for the metabolically active anagen hair bulb (Fischer et al. 2008). In a mouse model, melatonin was shown to promote hair regeneration via activation of the Wnt/β-catenin pathway by upregulating the release of Wnt3a and Wnt5a and downregulating SFRP2 in hair follicle stem cells, assessed via co-administration of the melatonin receptor antagonist luzindole (Niu et al. 2024).
- *Clinical data*: While melatonin's effects on sleep cycles are well documented, its role in hair loss treatments requires more comprehensive research. Early studies show promising results, particularly regarding its antioxidative and cytoprotective properties in protecting hair follicles from damage. However, large-scale clinical trials are necessary to conclusively determine its efficacy in managing AGA and other hair loss conditions. Though there is a paucity of randomized controlled trials evaluating the efficacy of melatonin in the treatment of alopecia, there is some clinical data that show promise. One randomized controlled trial compared the efficacy of a 0.1% melatonin solution applied topically to placebo in women experiencing androgenetic or diffuse alopecia. Melatonin was shown to significantly increase occipital anagen hair rate in addition to frontal hair growth in the melatonin group, demonstrating potential efficacy outside of male androgenetic alopecia (Fischer et al. 2004). Moreover, clinical data show excellent tolerability of topical melatonin, with no significant influence on endogenous serum melatonin levels, in addition to no local irritation reported, with some studies even reporting improvement of seborrhea and seborrheic dermatitis on the scalp following treatment with topical melatonin (Fischer et al. 2012).

Dietary Modifications for Hair Health

In addition to supplementation, dietary modifications can play a significant role in promoting hair health and supporting the efficacy of hair restoration treatments. Practitioners should encourage patients to adopt a balanced, nutrient-rich diet that includes:

1. *Adequate protein intake*: Hair is primarily composed of protein, and an adequate intake of high-quality protein sources, such as lean meats, fish, eggs, and plant-based proteins, is essential for hair growth and maintenance.

2. *Iron-rich foods*: To prevent iron deficiency anemia, which is associated with hair loss, patients should be encouraged to consume iron-rich foods, such as red meat, poultry, fish, leafy green vegetables, and legumes.
3. *Biotin-rich foods*: Foods high in biotin, such as eggs, nuts, seeds, and whole grains, can help to support healthy hair growth and improve hair thickness.
4. *Vitamin C-rich foods*: Vitamin C is necessary for the production of collagen, which provides structural support to hair follicles. Citrus fruits, berries, kiwi, and leafy green vegetables are excellent sources of vitamin C.
5. *Omega-3 fatty acids*: Omega-3 fatty acids, found in fatty fish, flaxseeds, chia seeds, and walnuts, have anti-inflammatory properties and may help to support hair follicle health.

In addition to promoting the consumption of nutrient-rich foods, practitioners should also advise patients to limit their intake of processed foods, refined sugars, and excessive amounts of caffeine and alcohol, as these may contribute to hair loss and impair the overall health of the scalp and hair follicles.

Lifestyle Interventions

Lifestyle factors can significantly impact hair health and the success of hair restoration treatments. Practitioners should encourage patients to adopt healthy lifestyle habits that support optimal hair growth, such as:

1. *Stress management*: Chronic stress can contribute to hair loss and impair the efficacy of hair restoration treatments. Patients should be encouraged to engage in stress-reducing activities, such as exercise, meditation, and deep breathing.
2. *Adequate sleep*: Insufficient sleep can disrupt the hair growth cycle and contribute to hair loss. Patients should be advised to prioritize sleep and aim for 7–9 hours of quality sleep per night.
3. *Gentle hair care practices*: Harsh hair care practices, such as excessive heat styling, tight hairstyles, and aggressive brushing, can damage hair follicles and contribute to hair loss. Patients should be educated on gentle hair care techniques, such as using a wide-toothed comb, air-drying hair, and avoiding tight hairstyles.
4. *Sun protection*: Excessive sun exposure can damage hair follicles and contribute to hair loss. Patients should be advised to protect their scalp and hair from the sun by wearing hats or using hair products with UV protection.

By addressing lifestyle factors that may contribute to hair loss, practitioners can help patients create a supportive environment for hair growth and enhance the outcomes of non-surgical hair restoration treatments.

Shampoo and Conditioner

Shampoos and conditioners play a crucial role in maintaining hair health and preventing the buildup of harmful pollutants and particulate matter on the scalp that may have a detrimental impact on hair health and growth. Scientifically, shampoos are primarily surfactant-based cleansers. Surfactants, such as sodium lauryl sulfate or sodium laureth sulfate, are amphiphilic molecules with hydrophilic (water-attracting) and lipophilic (oil-attracting) properties. These molecules effectively remove sebum, dirt, sweat, and environmental contaminants from the hair and scalp. However, these cleansing can also make many shampoos harsh and even damaging to hair.

Conditioners, in contrast, are formulated to counteract the harsh effects of cleansing and restore the hair's natural protective layer. They often contain cationic surfactants (e.g., behentrimonium chloride) that bind to the negatively charged surface of hair strands, reducing static and smoothing the cuticle. Other common ingredients include silicones (such as dimethicone) that form a protective layer on the hair shaft to enhance shine and reduce friction, emollients to provide hydration, and proteins to repair damaged keratin structures. The acidic pH of conditioners helps tighten the hair cuticle, locking in moisture and improving its resilience.

Some ingredients commonly used in shampoos and conditioners, namely phthalates, parabens, and sulfates, have detrimental effects on health and should be avoided. Sulfates bind to oil, grease, dirt, and fat and serve as effective cleansers of the scalp, prompting their widespread use in shampoos. Some sulfates, such as sodium lauryl sulfate, can exert an irritating effect on the scalp and can damage hair follicles (Monselise et al. 2015). Parabens are also frequently used in commercial shampoos and conditioners, serving a preservative function in these preparations. Finally, phthalates are also used in many shampoo and conditioner preparations as preservatives and to create a gel-like consistency in the products.

There are, however, many issues associated with exposure to these compounds that extend beyond hair and follicle health. These compounds are known endocrine disruptors. For example. Phthalates are known to result in altered androgen and estrogen response, spermatogenesis, and hormonal regulation (Chen et al. 2018) in addition to having negative impacts on skin, producing dermatological reactions and irritation to mucous membranes (Wang and Qian 2021). Parabens have similarly been implicated in the pathogenesis of endocrinological disruption, carcinogenesis, and dermatological issues (Fransway et al. 2019). As such, it is important to counsel patients on the importance of choosing personal care products, particularly shampoos, conditioners, and other hair serums and oils, that do not contain these compounds.

Conclusion

Nutritional and supplemental therapies are essential components of a comprehensive approach to non-surgical hair restoration. By addressing nutritional deficiencies, recommending evidence-based supplements, and promoting dietary modifications and healthy lifestyle habits, practitioners can support the overall health of the scalp and hair follicles, thereby enhancing the efficacy of other hair restoration treatments.

As with any therapeutic intervention, it is crucial for practitioners to individualize nutritional and supplemental recommendations based on each patient's unique needs, medical history, and treatment goals. By staying abreast of the latest research and best practices in nutritional and supplemental therapies for hair loss, practitioners can provide their patients with the most effective and evidence-based recommendations.

In the following chapters, we will explore advanced and emerging therapies in non-surgical hair restoration, including stem cell therapy, exosome therapy, and hormonal treatments. By integrating these cutting-edge approaches with the foundational strategies discussed in the previous chapters, practitioners can offer their patients the most comprehensive and individualized hair restoration plans, ultimately leading to optimal outcomes and patient satisfaction.

Chapter 11

Stem Cell Therapy

Julyssa A. Renteria and Robert Dorfman

Introduction

Stem cell therapy has garnered significant attention as a cutting-edge approach in non-surgical hair restoration, offering the potential to address hair loss through regenerative medicine. By leveraging the unique properties of stem cells, including their capacity for self-renewal and differentiation into specialized cell types, this therapy aims to rejuvenate damaged or dormant hair follicles and stimulate the growth of new, healthy hair. Current research has demonstrated the ability of stem cells to modulate perifollicular angiogenesis, secrete growth factors, and create a favorable microenvironment for hair regeneration.

This chapter will provide a comprehensive overview of stem cell therapy for hair restoration, focusing on the types of stem cells currently being explored, their mechanisms of action, and the evolving clinical applications. Additionally, emerging research and future directions will be discussed, including combination therapies, exosome-based approaches, and advancements in tissue engineering. By critically evaluating the evidence and understanding the practical aspects of stem cell therapy, practitioners can assess its role in their clinical practice and provide patients with informed, innovative options for managing hair loss.

Types of Stem Cells Used

Stem cells are unique in their ability to self-renew and differentiate into specialized cell types, making them a promising tool in regenerative medicine. In the context of hair restoration, they offer significant potential to enhance follicular regeneration and promote hair growth by leveraging their paracrine signaling capabilities and ability to influence key cellular pathways. Among the various types investigated, mesenchymal stem cells (MSCs), adipose-derived stem cells (ADSCs), and dermal papilla cells (DPCs) have emerged as leading candidates due to their accessibility, regenerative properties, and documented therapeutic efficacy. Each of these cell types plays a distinct role in addressing the complex pathophysiology of hair loss, whether by directly regenerating hair follicles, modulating the follicular microenvironment, or enhancing hair cycling through growth factor secretion and signaling pathway activation.

DOI: 10.1201/9781032726397-11

Mesenchymal Stem Cells (MSCs)

MSCs are multipotent stem cells capable of differentiating into various cell types, including those integral to hair follicle formation and maintenance. Derived from sources such as bone marrow, adipose tissue, and umbilical cord blood, MSCs have demonstrated significant promise in hair restoration therapies. Six months after stem cell therapy (SCT) injections, studies reported significant improvements in hair density and thickness, confirmed by immunostaining and digital dermoscopy, with the mean improvement rated as "very good" (Elmaadawi et al. 2018). No serious adverse events were observed, underscoring the safety profile of this therapy. MSCs promote hair growth through various mechanisms, such as activating the Wnt/β-catenin signaling pathway in DPCs, which enhances follicle regeneration, increases skin thickness, and prolongs the anagen phase of the hair cycle (Yan et al. 2024). Additionally, MSCs inhibit DPC apoptosis while promoting hair follicle stem cell (HFSC) proliferation, and umbilical cord-derived MSCs have shown the ability to protect against dexamethasone-induced apoptotic cell death in hair follicles (Bak et al. 2020).

Adipose-Derived Stem Cells (ADSCs)

ADSCs are a subtype of MSCs that can be easily obtained from adipose tissue through minimally invasive procedures such as liposuction. Their accessibility, abundance, and regenerative properties have made them a focus of research in hair restoration, particularly for treating resistant cases of alopecia areata (AA) and androgenetic alopecia (AGA). ADSCs have been shown to promote hair growth through the secretion of growth factors, including vascular endothelial growth factor (VEGF) and insulin-like growth factor-1 (IGF-1), which stimulate the proliferation and differentiation of hair follicle cells (Fukuoka and Suga 2015) (Figure 11.1). Recent advancements have

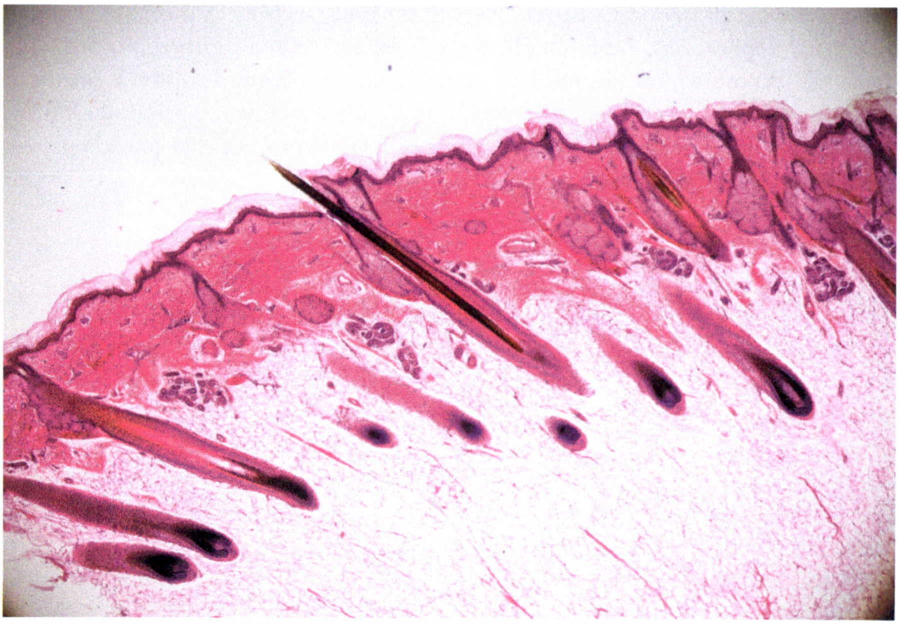

Figure 11.1 **Microscopy of hair follicles (from Shutterstock, under license).**

highlighted the potential of ADSCs and their derivatives in promoting hair regrowth. Conditioned media derived from ADSCs (ADSC-CM), when combined with fractional laser or microneedling, have demonstrated significant efficacy in improving hair regrowth in refractory AA cases. In a study by Lee et al. (2024), 64.3% of patients experienced more than 50% hair regrowth, with 42.9% achieving complete recovery. Similarly, exosomes derived from ADSCs (ADSC-Exos) have shown promise in enhancing DPC proliferation, migration, and reducing apoptosis. In mouse models, ADSC-Exos not only increased hair follicle density but also activated the Wnt/β-catenin signaling pathway, suggesting their utility in treating immune-mediated alopecia (Li 2022). Additionally, Liang et al. (2023) demonstrated that ADSC-Exos carrying miR-122-5p mitigated the inhibitory effects of dihydrotestosterone (DHT) on hair follicles by targeting the TGF-β1/SMAD3 signaling pathway. Other derivatives, such as stromal vascular fraction (SVF), have also shown effectiveness. Kang et al. (2022) conducted a systematic review, concluding that autologous SVF improved hair density and diameter in patients with non-scarring alopecia, including AGA and AA, without significant adverse events. Furthermore, studies by Anderi et al. (2018) demonstrated that autologous ADSVCs (adipose-derived stromal vascular cells) significantly improved hair density, quality, and regeneration in patients with AA.

Dermal Papilla Cells (DPCs)

DPCs are specialized mesenchymal cells located at the base of hair follicles that play a critical role in hair follicle morphogenesis and the regulation of hair growth cycles. Functioning as a signaling center, DPCs influence the activity of surrounding follicular cells through paracrine signaling, secreting key growth factors such as IGF-1, keratinocyte growth factor (KGF), and hepatocyte growth factor (HGF). These signaling molecules promote the proliferation and differentiation of epithelial stem cells, thereby supporting the development and cycling of hair follicles. Recent research has focused on new ways to utilize DPCs for hair restoration. Exosomes derived from DPCs have demonstrated the ability to enhance DPC and outer root sheath (ORS) cell proliferation, induce the anagen phase, and prolong its duration, effectively promoting hair regeneration (Kwack et al. 2019). Similarly, injectable platelet-rich fibrin (i-PRF) has shown promise in facilitating hair follicle regeneration by enhancing the proliferation, migration, and trichogenic inductivity of DPCs (Lu et al. 2021). Emerging technologies, such as sustained release systems, have expanded the potential applications of DPCs (Chen et al. 2020). For instance, encapsulation of DPC-derived extracellular vesicles (DP-EVs) in hydrogels like partially oxidized sodium alginate (OSA) significantly improves the stability and retention of EVs, leading to enhanced hair growth via upregulation of signaling molecules such as Wnt3a and β-catenin. Moreover, layer-by-layer (LBL) encapsulation techniques have been developed to deliver individual DPCs with cytokines, preserving their viability and functionality while promoting hair follicle regeneration (Lin et al. 2016). Non-invasive approaches such as electrical stimulation (ES) have shown the ability to restore the trichogenic activity of DPCs (Yan 2022). ES enhances trichogenic gene expression and improves the hair-inductive potential of DPCs, offering a novel and effective method for hair regenerative medicine.

The selection of stem cell types and therapeutic approaches for hair restoration must consider several factors, including the patient's underlying condition, the safety profile of the intervention, and the practical feasibility of the treatment. While MSCs, ADSCs, and DPCs have demonstrated efficacy in preclinical and clinical studies, the field remains in its infancy, with several challenges to address. Standardized protocols for cell isolation, preparation, and administration are essential to optimize therapeutic outcomes and ensure reproducibility. Additionally, further research is needed to fully elucidate the mechanisms by which these cells influence hair growth and to identify patient-specific factors that may predict treatment response. Despite these challenges, the potential of stem cell therapies to transform hair restoration is evident, offering hope for innovative and effective solutions for patients with hair loss.

Mechanisms and Clinical Applications

The mechanisms by which stem cells promote hair growth and regeneration are complex and multifaceted. Stem cells can exert their therapeutic effects through several key processes, including:

1. *Paracrine signaling*: Stem cells secrete a range of growth factors, cytokines, and extracellular vesicles that influence the surrounding follicular environment. These signaling molecules stimulate the proliferation and differentiation of hair follicle cells, enhance angiogenesis to improve follicular blood supply, and regulate inflammation. This process creates a favorable niche for hair growth, with evidence demonstrating that paracrine signaling is central to the repair and regeneration of damaged hair follicles (Chen et al. 2020).
2. *Cell differentiation*: Stem cells have the ability to differentiate into specialized cells essential for hair follicle function, such as keratinocytes and dermal papilla cells. By replenishing the pool of these specialized cells, stem cells regenerate damaged or dormant hair follicles and restore their ability to support hair growth.
3. *Immunomodulation*: Chronic inflammation is a key contributor to hair loss in conditions like AGA and AA. Stem cells help regulate the inflammatory response by reducing pro-inflammatory cytokine levels and modulating immune cell activity. This immunomodulatory effect mitigates inflammation, creating a healthier environment for hair follicles and promoting their recovery.

Clinical Applications

The clinical applications of stem cell therapy in hair restoration are rapidly evolving (Gentile and Garcovich 2019). Currently, several approaches are being investigated.

Autologous Stem Cell Transplantation

This approach involves harvesting stem cells from the patient's own tissues, such as adipose tissue or bone marrow, and reintroducing them into the scalp to regenerate hair follicles. By modulating the follicular microenvironment and promoting cellular proliferation, this has shown promise in improving hair density and follicular health, particularly in patients with advanced AGA. The clinical safety and efficacy of autologous stem cell transplantation have been demonstrated in multiple studies (Gasteratos et al. 2024). Fukuoka and Suga (2015) reported significant improvements in hair density and thickness in patients treated with ADSCs. Similarly, Gan et al. (2024) conducted a trial involving 50 patients with advanced AGA who received autologous hair follicle MSC suspensions. The study found notable increases in terminal hair proportion and hair shaft diameter within 1 month, with effects persisting up to 3 months. These improvements were particularly evident in miniaturized hair follicles with diameters under 60 μm. Another study evaluated autologous SVF therapy in nine patients with AGA, reporting significant increases in hair density at 3 and 6 months post-transplantation compared to untreated areas. Although a rise in hair thickness was observed, it was not statistically significant. In a larger multicentric study, Gentile et al. (2024) treated 60 patients with autologous micrografts containing human follicle mesenchymal stem cells (HF-MSCs). Their findings demonstrated significant improvements in hair density (28 ± 4 hairs/cm² in females and 30 ± 5 hairs/cm² in males) at 12 months, with extracellular vesicles (EVs) playing a pivotal role in enhancing the regenerative process. Autologous stem cell transplantation is generally safe and well tolerated, with minimal adverse effects reported across studies (Anderi et al. 2018). The use of autologous cells minimizes the risk of immune rejection and related complications, making it an attractive option for patients.

Allogeneic Stem Cell Transplantation

This approach involves the use of stem cells derived from donor sources such as umbilical cord blood or placental tissue. These cells can be expanded in vitro and used to treat multiple patients, making this approach a scalable and potentially transformative option in regenerative medicine. A study by Oh et al. (2020) demonstrated promising results in the treatment of AGA using umbilical cord blood-derived MSCs, with improvements observed in hair density. In addition to hair restoration, allogeneic stem cells show potential for treating autoimmune-related hair loss, such as AA and alopecia universalis. Immune system replacement through allogeneic hematopoietic stem cell transplantation (HSCT) replaces the recipient's immune system with that of a healthy donor. This process has been shown to induce remission in autoimmune conditions. In one case, a patient with alopecia universalis experienced complete hair regrowth following allogeneic HSCT, as the new immune system lacked the autoreactive components that previously attacked the patient's hair follicles (Seifert et al. 2005). Beyond immune system replacement, allogeneic MSCs also exhibit significant immunomodulatory properties (Kim et al. 2022). MSCs derived from healthy donors can suppress the activation of proinflammatory T cells (Th1 and Th17) while enhancing regulatory T cells (Tregs), thereby promoting immune tolerance and reducing inflammation. This effect is particularly relevant in AA, where the immune privilege of hair follicles is often compromised.

Stem Cell-Derived Growth Factors

Stem cells can be cultured in vitro to produce a conditioned medium (CM) rich in growth factors and cytokines that promote hair growth. This conditioned medium can be applied topically or injected into the scalp (Oh et al. 2024), offering a non-surgical approach to enhance follicular regeneration and hair density. The growth factors present in stem cell-derived CM and exosomes stimulate DPCs and HFSCs, key players in hair follicle development and cycling. Notable growth factors include insulin-like growth factor (IGF), platelet-derived growth factor (PDGF), basic fibroblast growth factor (bFGF), and Wnt7a. These factors collectively promote cellular proliferation, inhibit apoptosis, and induce the anagen phase of hair follicles, creating a favorable environment for hair regrowth. Evidence supports the efficacy of stem cell-derived CM in increasing hair density and thickness. For instance, a meta-analysis of clinical trials demonstrated significant improvements in hair density (mean difference [MD]: 14.93, 95% CI: 10.20–19.67) and hair thickness (MD: 18.67, 95% CI: 2.75–34.59) in patients treated with CM (Chien 2024). Moreover, ADSC-Exos have been shown to counteract the inhibitory effects of DHT on hair follicles by modulating the TGF-β1/SMAD3 signaling pathway promoting hair follicle regeneration.

While these clinical applications show promise, it is important to note that stem cell therapy for hair restoration is still in its early stages, and further research is needed to establish its long-term safety and efficacy. Practitioners should keep abreast of the latest developments in this field and carefully consider the evidence when incorporating stem cell therapy into their hair restoration practice.

Practical Applications of Stem Cell Therapy in Hair Restoration

Stem cell-based treatments for hair restoration require careful handling and administration to ensure their efficacy and minimize potential complications. The following outlines the key steps and considerations involved in the use of stem cells for clinical hair restoration.

Preparation and Handling

Stem cells used for hair restoration are typically cryopreserved to maintain their viability and potency. Proper storage at ultra-low temperatures (–80°C or below) is essential to prevent cellular degradation. Before administration, the stem cells are thawed under controlled conditions to preserve their functionality. Any deviation in storage or thawing protocols can compromise the effectiveness of the treatment.

Administration Techniques

The thawed stem cell product is often delivered to the scalp through microneedling or direct injection into the dermis of the affected areas. Microneedling enhances the penetration of growth factors and cytokines into the scalp, while also stimulating local blood flow and promoting a regenerative environment. In some cases, stem cells are combined with a carrier medium, such as a hydrogel or platelet-rich plasma (PRP), to improve their retention and distribution.

Patient Counseling

When counseling patients about stem cell therapy for hair restoration, physicians must provide clear, comprehensive information to ensure informed decision-making. Begin by educating patients about the basics of stem cell therapy. Explain that the treatment leverages stem cells sourced from adipose tissue, bone marrow, or umbilical cord blood, which release growth factors and cytokines to stimulate hair follicle regeneration and enhance the hair growth cycle. It is essential to emphasize that this therapy is not yet considered a standard of care, and while clinical studies have shown promising results, it remains an evolving field with variable outcomes.

Setting realistic expectations is critical. Physicians should outline the therapy's goals, such as increasing hair density, improving hair thickness, and enhancing overall hair quality. It is important to clarify that the treatment aims to slow the progression of hair loss and promote regrowth rather than fully restoring preexisting hair density. Patients should also be informed that optimal results often require multiple sessions spaced several months apart, depending on the severity of their hair loss and their individual response to treatment.

Patients must also understand the potential risks and safety profile of stem cell therapy. While the treatment is generally well tolerated, localized side effects such as edema, erythema, or minor discomfort at the injection site may occur. With autologous stem cell treatments, the risk of immune rejection is minimal, but rare complications, such as contamination or immune reactions, may arise with allogeneic therapies. Physicians should also explain that individual responses to treatment can vary based on the cause of hair loss, biological factors, and the stage of alopecia.

The treatment process itself should be discussed in detail. Stem cells or their derivatives, such as conditioned medium or exosomes, are typically injected into the scalp via intradermal injections. To enhance the regenerative effects, techniques such as microneedling or fractional laser therapy may be combined with stem cell delivery. After treatment, patients should follow specific post-procedure guidelines, including avoiding hair washing for 24 hours, refraining from using NSAIDs for 48–72 hours to allow natural inflammatory processes to occur, and elevating the head during sleep to minimize swelling. Patients should also be advised to protect their scalp from direct sunlight for several days to prevent irritation.

Physicians should highlight the current evidence base to build patient confidence while also acknowledging its limitations. Clinical studies have demonstrated that autologous ADSCs and exosomes can significantly increase hair density and thickness in conditions like AGA and AA. However, it is important to note that further large-scale studies are needed to establish standardized protocols and determine the durability of these outcomes.

Finally, obtaining informed consent is essential. Physicians should ensure that patients fully understand the experimental nature of stem cell therapy, the potential benefits and risks, and alternative treatment options such as minoxidil, finasteride, or PRP therapy. Discuss the financial implications, as stem cell therapies are not typically covered by insurance, and encourage patients to ask questions to address any concerns.

Post-Treatment Care

To optimize treatment outcomes and minimize complications, the following post-treatment guidelines should be provided to patients:

- *Avoid anti-inflammatory medications*: Patients should refrain from using NSAIDs for at least 48–72 hours following treatment, as these may interfere with the inflammatory and healing processes that are integral to the therapy's efficacy.
- *Delay hair washing*: Patients should avoid washing their hair until the day after treatment to allow the scalp to heal and the stem cells to integrate into the treated areas.
- *Head positioning*: It is advisable to keep the head elevated while sleeping on the night after treatment to reduce swelling and improve blood circulation to the scalp.
- *Sun protection*: Patients should avoid direct sun exposure to the treated areas for several days to minimize irritation and potential damage to the scalp.

Monitoring and Follow-Up

Patients should return for follow-up evaluations to assess the response to treatment and monitor for any adverse effects. Physicians may recommend multiple sessions spaced several weeks apart to achieve optimal results, depending on the severity of hair loss and the patient's response to the initial treatment.

Current Research and Future Directions

Stem cell therapy for hair restoration is an evolving field with ongoing research aimed at refining its therapeutic applications. Some of the current research directions and future prospects include:

1. *Genetically modified stem cells*: Genetic modifications are enhancing the regenerative potential of stem cells, particularly for patients with AGA and AA. For example, mesenchymal stem cells derived from amniotic fluid and genetically engineered to overexpress the Nanog gene have demonstrated the ability to enhance dermal papilla cell activity, promote follicular regeneration, and boost secretion of growth factors such as IGF, PDGF, bFGF, and Wnt7a (Park et al. 2019). Similarly, CRISPR/Cas9 gene-editing technology has been used to knock out the DKK1 gene in ADSCs (Choi et al. 2024). This modification improves cell motility, reduces senescence, and activates the Wnt signaling pathway, resulting in more robust hair growth compared to unmodified ADSCs.
2. *Combination therapies*: Combining stem cell therapy with other hair restoration treatments, such as PRP, microneedling, or low-level laser therapy, may provide synergistic effects and enhance treatment outcomes (Stevens et al. 2018). Research is ongoing to explore the optimal combinations and protocols for these combination therapies.
3. *Tissue engineering*: The development of bioengineered hair follicles using stem cells and biomaterials is an exciting prospect in hair restoration. This approach involves creating three-dimensional, functional hair follicles in vitro that can be transplanted into the scalp. While still in the early stages of research, tissue engineering holds promise for the treatment of severe hair loss and the creation of personalized hair restoration solutions (Abaci et al. 2018).
4. *Clinical trial design*: Improving the design and standardization of clinical trials is crucial for advancing the field of stem cell therapy for hair restoration. Future studies should focus on larger, well-controlled trials with longer follow-up periods to better assess the safety, efficacy, and long-term outcomes of stem cell therapies (Gentile and Garcovich 2019).

To fully integrate these innovations into clinical practice, further research is needed to standardize protocols and conduct large-scale trials. As these technologies mature, they hold promise to expand the options available for patients with hair loss.

Conclusion

Stem cell therapy is emerging as a transformative approach in non-surgical hair restoration, offering the ability to regenerate hair follicles, stimulate hair growth, and potentially reverse hair loss. By leveraging the unique properties of stem cells, such as self-renewal, differentiation, and the secretion of bioactive molecules, this therapy provides a regenerative and targeted alternative to traditional treatments for hair loss.

Although still in its early stages, current evidence indicates that stem cell therapy holds considerable promise for patients with androgenetic alopecia and other forms of hair loss. Current research is shedding light on its mechanisms of action, refining treatment protocols, and exploring innovative strategies such as exosome-based therapies, genetic modifications, and tissue engineering. These advancements suggest a future where stem cell therapy could redefine the landscape of hair restoration.

However, practitioners must approach stem cell therapy with caution, grounding their clinical decisions in robust evidence. Questions about long-term safety, efficacy, and the standardization of treatment protocols remain unanswered. As with any emerging therapy, it is essential to balance innovation with a commitment to patient safety and evidence-based practice.

By staying informed about the latest developments, critically appraising research, and collaborating with experts in the field, practitioners can responsibly integrate stem cell therapy into their clinical practice. This evolving treatment modality holds the potential to offer patients a cutting-edge solution to hair loss, ultimately improving their quality of life and confidence. As advancements continue, stem cell therapy may pave the way for a new era in hair restoration, benefiting countless individuals worldwide.

Chapter 12

Exosome Therapy

Julyssa A. Renteria and Robert Dorfman

Introduction

Exosome therapy is a rapidly emerging treatment in non-surgical hair restoration, offering a new approach to addressing hair loss (Kost et al. 2022; Gupta et al. 2023). Exosomes are small extracellular vesicles secreted by cells that carry bioactive molecules, including growth factors, cytokines, and microRNAs, which play a key role in cellular communication and tissue repair. In hair restoration, exosomes are used to enhance follicular function, stimulate hair growth, and improve scalp health by delivering these bioactive molecules directly to hair follicles. This chapter explores the therapeutic potential of exosome therapy, focusing on its mechanisms of action, clinical applications, and safety profile. It also examines current evidence supporting its use and highlights emerging research aimed at optimizing its efficacy. By understanding the practical aspects of exosome therapy, practitioners can evaluate its role in their clinical practice and consider its integration as a promising tool for managing hair loss.

Understanding Exosomes

Exosomes are small extracellular vesicles, typically measuring 30 to 150 nm in diameter, enclosed by a lipid bilayer. Secreted by various cell types, including stem cells, exosomes play a pivotal role in intercellular communication, facilitating the transfer of bioactive molecules such as proteins, lipids, nucleic acids (e.g., mRNA and microRNA), and signaling molecules. These vesicles influence recipient cell behavior and function, making them highly relevant in regenerative medicine (Raposo and Stoorvogel 2013). The unique properties of exosomes provide several advantages over traditional cell-based therapies:

- *Cell-free therapy*: Exosomes can be isolated and purified from cell cultures, offering a cell-free approach that reduces risks associated with cell transplantation, such as immune rejection and tumorigenicity.
- *Stability and scalability*: Exosomes demonstrate enhanced stability compared to cells, retaining their biological activity during extended storage. This stability supports the development of off-the-shelf, scalable therapies that are easily transportable and ready for use.

DOI: 10.1201/9781032726397-12

- *Targeted delivery*: Exosomes exhibit natural targeting capabilities, interacting with specific receptors on recipient cells to deliver bioactive molecules directly. This precision minimizes off-target effects while enhancing therapeutic efficacy.
- *Biocompatibility*: Derived from natural sources, exosomes share compositional similarities with the extracellular matrix, resulting in high biocompatibility and a low risk of adverse reactions.

In hair restoration, the therapeutic potential of exosomes lies in their ability to deliver concentrated growth factors, cytokines, and signaling molecules to hair follicles. This targeted delivery stimulates the proliferation and differentiation of hair follicle stem cells, enhances angiogenesis, and modulates the inflammatory response in the scalp, creating an optimal environment for hair regeneration (Hu et al. 2024). See Figure 12.1.

Therapeutic Potential and Clinical Applications

The use of exosome therapy in hair restoration is a rapidly evolving field, with promising preclinical and early clinical evidence supporting its therapeutic potential. Exosomes derived from various cell types, such as mesenchymal stem cells (MSCs), adipose-derived stem cells (ADSCs), and dermal papilla cells (DPCs), have been investigated for their ability to promote hair growth and regeneration. See Figures 12.2 and 12.3.

Preclinical Studies

Building on the foundational principles of stem cells discussed in the previous chapter, exosome therapy leverages cell-derived vesicles to achieve regenerative outcomes without the need for direct cell transplantation. Exosomes from various cellular sources have shown significant promise in

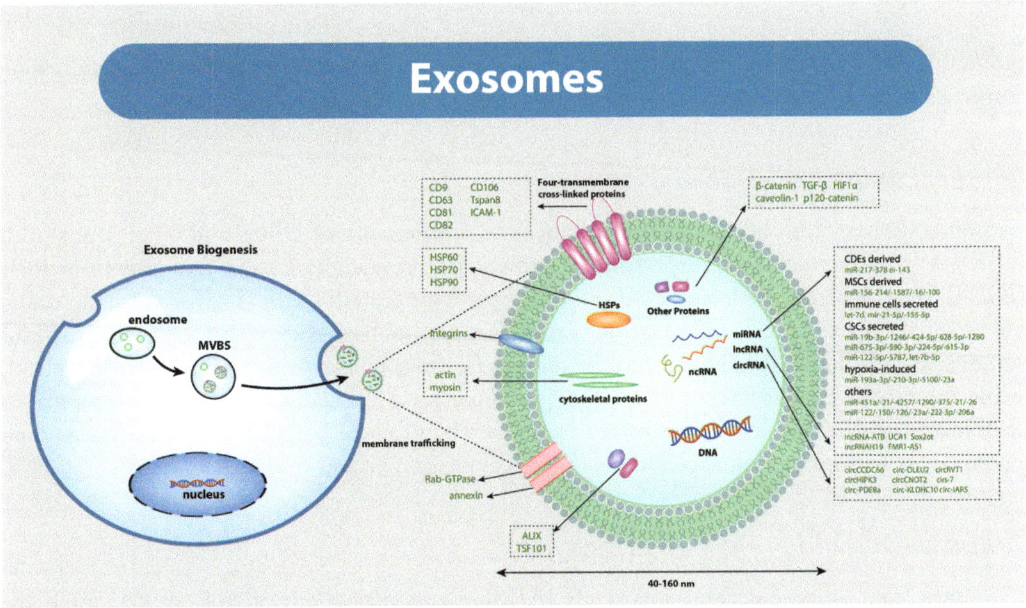

Figure 12.1 Structure, biogenesis, and function of exosomes—small extracellular vesicles (30–150 nm) enclosed by a lipid bilayer (from Shutterstock, under license).

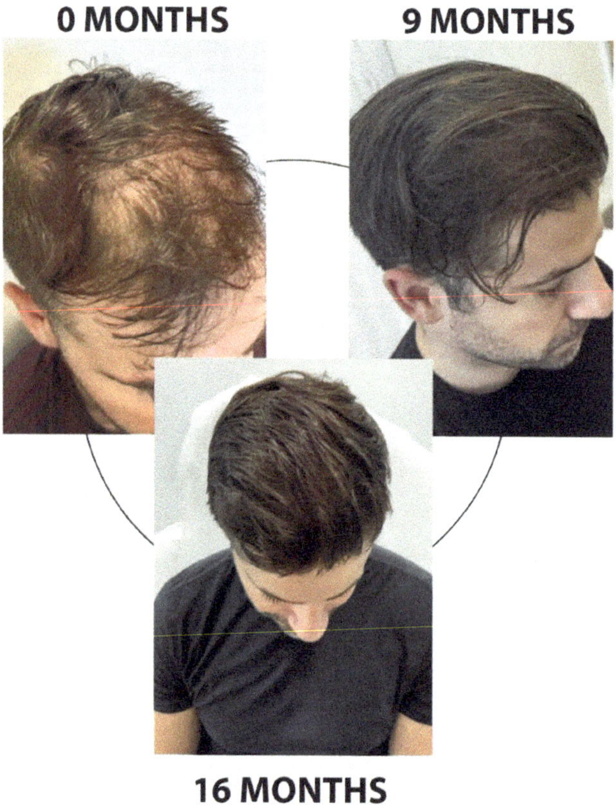

Figure 12.2 The hair restoration process at 0 months, 9 months, and 16 months following exosome therapy.

promoting hair growth and regenerating hair follicles, offering a cell-free approach to addressing alopecia areata (AA), androgenetic alopecia (AGA), and other forms of hair loss.

Dermal Papilla Cell-Derived Exosomes

Exosomes derived from human DPCs enhance the proliferation of DPCs and outer root sheath (ORS) cells by increasing the expression of growth factors such as insulin-like growth factor-1 (IGF-1), keratinocyte growth factor (KGF), and hepatocyte growth factor (HGF). These molecules are essential for hair follicle regeneration. Preclinical studies have shown that DPC-derived exosomes can transition hair follicles from the telogen (resting) phase to the anagen (growth) phase, while also prolonging the anagen phase in mouse models. Additionally, when used in conjunction with mouse epidermal cells, these exosomes promoted hair follicle neogenesis, demonstrating their potential for hair restoration applications (Kwack et al. 2019; Zhou et al. 2018).

Adipose-Derived Stem Cell Exosomes

Exosomes from adipose-derived stem cells (ADSC-Exos) play a critical role in activating the Wnt/β-catenin signaling pathway, a key regulator of hair follicle regeneration. These exosomes

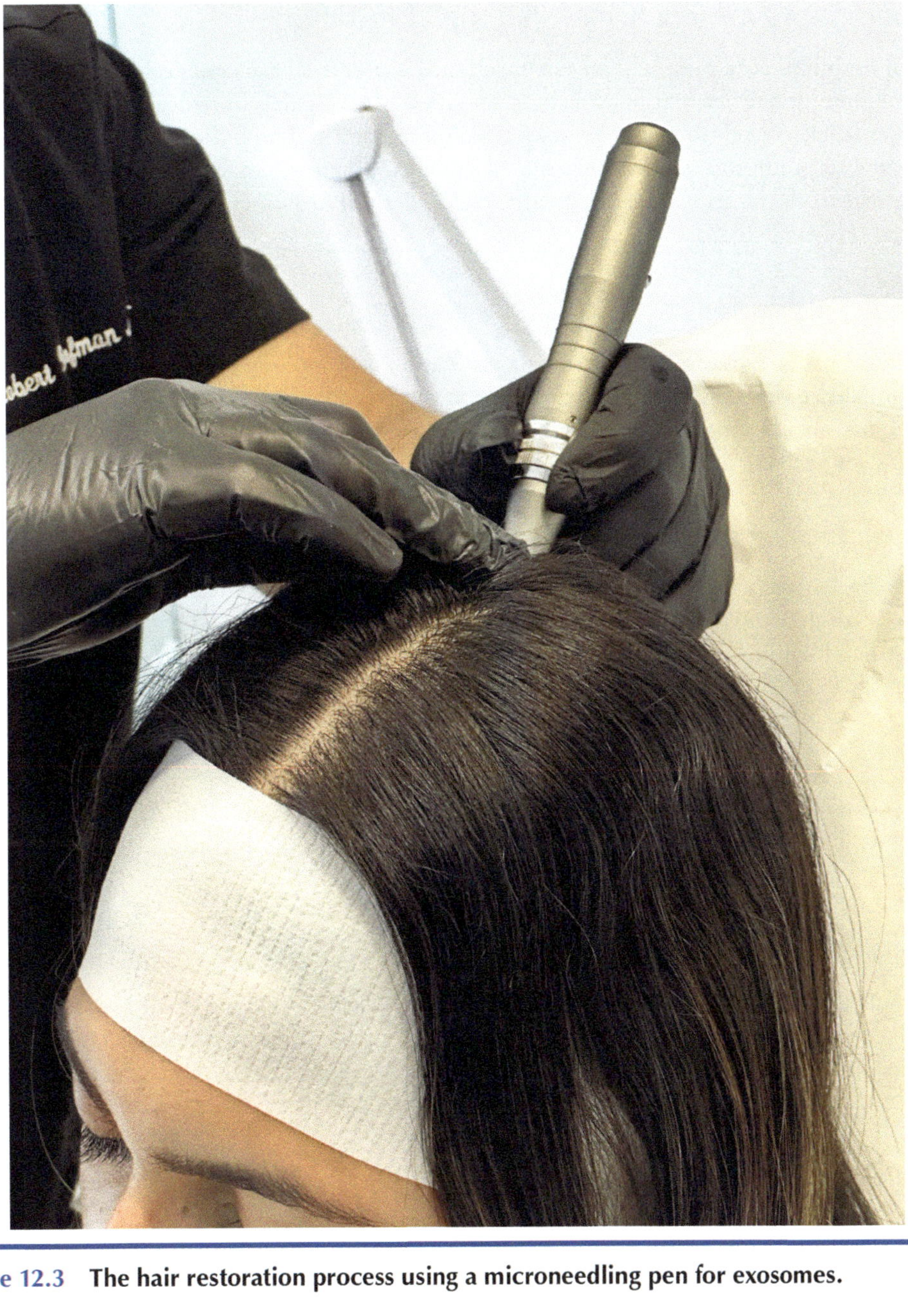

Figure 12.3 **The hair restoration process using a microneedling pen for exosomes.**

counteract the inhibitory effects of dihydrotestosterone (DHT) on hair follicles, promoting dermal papilla cell proliferation, migration, and differentiation. Preclinical models have reported significant improvements in hair growth, increased follicle density, and dermal thickening following treatment with ADSC-Exos. Furthermore, these exosomes modulate pathways such as miR-22 and TNF-α, enhancing their regenerative effects (Li et al. 2022; Tang et al. 2023).

Umbilical Cord Mesenchymal Stem Cell Exosomes

Human umbilical cord mesenchymal stem cell (uMSC)-derived exosomes offer a high-yield, efficient solution for hair restoration. Preclinical studies in AA models have demonstrated that these exosomes accelerate hair follicular keratinocyte proliferation and migration, resulting in improved hair regrowth. Additional studies have shown significant increases in follicle density, hair growth, and dermal thickness in mice treated with uMSC-derived exosomes, highlighting their clinical potential (Hu et al. 2024).

Clinical Applications

The clinical use of exosome therapy in hair restoration is in its early stages, but emerging studies have provided promising evidence supporting its safety and efficacy in treating AGA and other forms of hair loss. A range of clinical trials and case studies highlight the potential of exosomes to stimulate hair growth and improve hair density and thickness (Queen and Avram 2024).

Adipose-Derived Stem Cell Exosomes

A study by Park et al. (2022) retrospectively analyzed 39 patients treated with topical ADSC exosomes combined with microneedling. Patients underwent weekly sessions for 12 weeks and demonstrated significant increases in hair density and thickness, though some reported mild discomfort during the microneedling process.

Umbilical Cord Mesenchymal Stem Cell Exosomes

A prospective study by Ersan et al. (2024) treated 30 male patients with AGA using foreskin-derived MSC exosomes. The study reported a statistically significant increase in hair density at 12 weeks, with no adverse reactions.

Comparisons with Platelet-Rich Plasma (PRP)

In a comparative case series by Hassan et al. (2024), patients receiving a single session of human-derived exosome therapy demonstrated superior and longer-lasting improvements in hair density and thickness compared to those undergoing five to six sessions of PRP over 6 months. This finding highlights the potential of exosome therapy as an efficient alternative to traditional treatments.

Specialized Applications

In a unique approach, Norooznezhad et al. (2023) reported on a patient with chemotherapy-induced alopecia treated with placental MSC-derived exosome-enriched extracellular vesicles. The patient received injections every 4 weeks for 3 months and achieved complete regrowth of terminal hair, with no adverse events reported.

While these studies highlight the therapeutic potential of exosome therapy for hair restoration, the field faces several challenges that must be addressed. Variability in exosome sources, isolation methods, and dosing protocols complicates the standardization and comparison of results across studies. Furthermore, exosome therapies currently lack FDA approval, necessitating rigorous clinical trials to establish their safety, efficacy, and quality control. These challenges will be discussed further in the following section.

Safety

The safety of exosome therapy is a critical consideration for both practitioners and patients. While this treatment has shown promise in promoting hair growth, it remains an experimental approach with limited long-term safety data. Early clinical evidence suggests that exosome therapy is generally well-tolerated, with a favorable safety profile when applied locally or topically.

Key Safety Features

1. *Non-immunogenic and biocompatible*: Exosomes are naturally derived extracellular vesicles with a lipid bilayer structure similar to the extracellular matrix. Their non-immunogenic nature reduces the risk of immune rejection, making them suitable for allogeneic (donor-derived) use.
2. *Minimal side effects*: Clinical studies have reported mild, transient side effects, such as redness, swelling, or itching at the injection site, which typically resolve within a few days. For example, in a study of ADSC-Exos for AGA, no severe adverse events were reported, and participants experienced significant increases in hair density and high satisfaction ratings (Lee et al. 2024). Similarly, a trial involving foreskin-derived mesenchymal stromal cell exosomes showed statistically significant hair density improvements at 4 and 12 weeks post-treatment without complications (Ersan et al. 2024).
3. *Systematic review findings*: A systematic review and meta-analysis of clinical trials assessing human extracellular vesicle-based therapies, including exosomes, found a low incidence of serious adverse events (0.7%) and general adverse events (4.4%) (Van Delen et al. 2024). These results reinforce the treatment's overall safety while emphasizing the importance of rigorous quality control and long-term monitoring.

Potential Risks and Uncertainties

Despite its promising safety profile, exosome therapy carries potential risks that require careful consideration:

- *Serious adverse events*: Rare but documented risks include allergic reactions, infections, thrombosis, and organ toxicity (Queen and Avram 2024). Additionally, concerns about tumorigenesis—exosomes potentially stimulating the growth of undetected cancerous cells—underscore the need for thorough patient screening. Patients with a history of cancer or active skin cancer in the treatment area should not undergo exosome therapy.
- *Regulatory oversight*: The US FDA has not approved exosome therapy for hair restoration and currently recommends its use only as a topical application. Challenges such as variability in exosome sources, manufacturing inconsistencies, and the lack of standardized purification and storage protocols hinder regulatory approval.
- *Long-term safety*: While short-term results are encouraging, long-term safety data are limited, necessitating further investigation into potential complications such as immune rejection, autoimmune reactions, cytokine release syndrome, and neurological effects.

Larger, well-controlled clinical trials with extended follow-up are essential to validate the safety, optimize protocols, and ensure consistent quality. For now, exosome therapy remains an experimental yet exciting frontier in the field of regenerative medicine for hair restoration.

Practical Applications of Exosome Therapy in Hair Restoration

Preparation and Handling

Exosomes used for hair restoration are typically cryopreserved to maintain their stability and biological activity. Proper storage at ultra-low temperatures (–80°C or below) is essential to prevent degradation of the bioactive molecules contained within. Before administration, exosomes are thawed under controlled conditions to preserve their functionality. The recommended thawing process involves placing the frozen exosome preparation at 4°C (refrigerator temperature) or on ice for 30–60 minutes, depending on the volume. This gradual thawing minimizes the risk of temperature shock, which can compromise the lipid bilayer or degrade the bioactive molecules. Direct heat sources, such as warm water baths or room temperature thawing, should be avoided. After thawing, the exosome solution should be gently mixed by inverting the container or lightly pipetting to ensure homogeneity without disrupting the vesicle membranes. It is crucial to use the exosome preparation immediately after thawing to maintain its biological activity. If immediate use is not feasible, the solution can be kept on ice for a few hours, but repeated freeze–thaw cycles must be avoided as they significantly degrade the exosomes' therapeutic properties. Any deviation in storage or thawing protocols can compromise the efficacy of the treatment.

Administration Techniques

Exosomes are commonly administered to the scalp via microneedling or direct intradermal injections. Microneedling creates microchannels in the scalp, enhancing the absorption and penetration of exosomes into the dermis. Additionally, it stimulates local blood flow and triggers a regenerative response, complementing the therapeutic effects of exosomes. Exosomes can also be directly injected into areas of hair thinning or loss. This targeted delivery method ensures that the bioactive molecules are concentrated in the areas requiring regeneration. In some cases, exosomes are combined with other therapies, such as PRP or growth factor-enriched hydrogels, to enhance retention and synergistic effects.

Patient Counseling

Effective patient counseling is essential to ensure informed decision-making and to set appropriate expectations for exosome therapy in hair restoration. Physicians should begin by explaining the treatment's experimental nature, emphasizing that exosomes are cell-derived vesicles containing growth factors, cytokines, and microRNAs that promote hair follicle regeneration and modulate the hair growth cycle. It is important to highlight that exosome therapy is not FDA approved for hair restoration and remains an evolving field. Patients should be informed of potential benefits, such as increased hair density and improved hair quality, while understanding that individual results may vary and multiple sessions may be required for optimal outcomes. Thorough screening is critical to identify contraindications; for instance, patients with a history of cancer or active skin cancer in the treatment area should be excluded due to the potential risks associated with growth factor stimulation. By providing clear, comprehensive information, physicians can help patients make confident, well-informed decisions about pursuing this treatment.

Post-Treatment Care

Proper post-treatment care is essential to optimize results and minimize complications.

- *Hair washing*: Patients should avoid washing their hair until the day after treatment to allow the exosomes to integrate into the scalp.
- *Anti-inflammatory medications*: Advise patients to refrain from using NSAIDs for 48–72 hours, as these may interfere with the natural inflammatory processes that contribute to the therapy's effectiveness.
- *Head elevation*: Recommend keeping the head elevated while sleeping on the night following treatment to reduce swelling and promote blood circulation to the scalp.
- *Sun protection*: Patients should avoid direct sun exposure to the treated areas for several days to minimize irritation and potential damage.

Monitoring and Follow-Up

Patients should return for follow-up evaluations to assess their response to treatment and monitor for any adverse effects. Multiple sessions may be recommended, spaced several weeks apart, depending on the severity of hair loss and individual response to the therapy.

Conclusion

As we have discussed in this chapter, exosome therapy offers a new, cell-free approach to non-surgical hair restoration, leveraging the regenerative potential of bioactive molecules to stimulate hair growth and improve follicle function. Emerging evidence highlights its ability to enhance hair density, promote follicular regeneration, and improve scalp health, making it a promising option for patients seeking innovative treatments. While the safety profile of exosome therapy appears favorable, it remains an experimental modality requiring further investigation. Challenges such as the lack of standardized protocols and long-term data must be addressed to fully realize its clinical potential. As research progresses and the field evolves, exosome therapy could become a valuable addition to the toolkit for managing hair loss. By staying informed about advancements and maintaining a cautious, evidence-based approach, practitioners can responsibly evaluate the role of exosome therapy in their practice. This treatment represents a significant step forward in hair restoration, offering new possibilities for patients and paving the way for continued innovation in the field.

Chapter 13

Patient Evaluation and Diagnosis

Julyssa A. Renteria and Robert Dorfman

Introduction

Thorough patient evaluation and accurate diagnosis are fundamental to the success of non-surgical hair restoration treatments. Each patient's hair loss is unique, influenced by factors such as medical history, genetic predisposition, lifestyle, and personal treatment goals. A detailed assessment allows practitioners to identify the underlying causes of hair loss, determine its severity, and tailor treatment strategies to achieve the best possible outcomes. This chapter explores the essential elements of patient evaluation, including comprehensive history taking, thorough clinical examination, and the utilization of advanced diagnostic tools and tests. It emphasizes the importance of integrating these insights into personalized treatment plans that align with each patient's needs and expectations. By refining their approach to patient evaluation and diagnosis, practitioners can deliver targeted and effective non-surgical hair restoration solutions, ultimately enhancing patient satisfaction and clinical success.

History Taking and Clinical Examination

The foundation of patient evaluation in non-surgical hair restoration is a thorough history taking and clinical examination. This process allows practitioners to gather essential information about the patient's hair loss journey, identify potential contributing factors, and assess the overall health and condition of the scalp and hair.

History Taking

A comprehensive patient history should cover the following key areas:

1. *Onset and progression of hair loss*: Patients should be asked about when they first noticed hair loss, the pattern and rate of progression, and any fluctuations in hair shedding or thinning over time. This information can help to differentiate between acute and chronic hair loss conditions and identify potential triggers or exacerbating factors.

DOI: 10.1201/9781032726397-13

2. *Family history of hair loss*: Inquiring about a family history of hair loss can provide insights into the patient's genetic predisposition to conditions such as androgenetic alopecia. This information can also guide the practitioner in setting realistic expectations for treatment outcomes and long-term management strategies.
3. *Medical history and medications*: A review of the patient's medical history, including chronic illnesses, autoimmune disorders, and endocrine abnormalities, can help to identify potential systemic causes of hair loss. It is also essential to inquire about the use of medications, as certain drugs, such as chemotherapeutic agents, anticoagulants, and hormone therapies, can contribute to hair loss.
4. *Nutritional status and dietary habits*: Assessing the patient's nutritional status and dietary habits can help to identify potential deficiencies or imbalances that may contribute to hair loss. Patients should be asked about their typical diet, any restrictive eating patterns, and the use of dietary supplements.
5. *Hair care practices and styling habits*: Discussing the patient's hair care practices and styling habits can provide insights into potential sources of mechanical or chemical damage to the hair. Patients should be asked about their use of heat styling tools, chemical treatments, and tight hairstyles, as these can contribute to hair breakage and traction alopecia.
6. *Psychosocial impact of hair loss*: Hair loss can have a significant impact on a patient's self-image, confidence, and overall quality of life. It is important to ask about the psychosocial effects of hair loss and assess the patient's motivation for seeking treatment. This information can help practitioners to provide appropriate emotional support and set realistic expectations for treatment outcomes.

Clinical Examination

A thorough clinical examination of the scalp and hair is essential for accurately diagnosing the type and extent of hair loss. The examination should include the following key components:

1. *Visual inspection*: The scalp and hair should be visually inspected under good lighting to assess the pattern and distribution of hair loss. Practitioners should note the presence of any visible thinning, widening of the part line, or recession of the hairline. The examination should also include an assessment of the hair shaft quality, noting any signs of breakage, thinning, or variation in thickness.
2. *Trichoscopy*: Trichoscopy, also known as dermoscopy of the scalp, is a non-invasive diagnostic tool that allows for the magnified visualization of the scalp and hair follicles (Figure 13.1). Using a handheld dermatoscope or a video trichoscope (Figure 13.2), practitioners can assess the density and diameter of hair follicles, identify miniaturization, and detect any signs of scalp inflammation or scarring. This diagnostic tool provides valuable insights into the underlying cause of hair loss and will help guide treatment decisions.
3. *Hair pull test*: The hair pull test is a simple clinical test used to assess the presence and severity of active hair shedding. The practitioner gently grasps a small bundle of hair (approximately 50–60 hairs) and applies gentle traction. The number of hairs that come out with each pull is counted and recorded. A positive hair pull test, typically defined as more than 10% of the grasped hairs coming out, can indicate active telogen effluvium or other forms of excessive shedding.
4. *Scalp biopsy*: In certain cases, a scalp biopsy may be necessary to confirm the diagnosis or rule out other potential causes of hair loss, such as scarring alopecia or alopecia areata. A punch biopsy of the scalp, typically 4–6 mm in diameter, is performed under local anesthesia

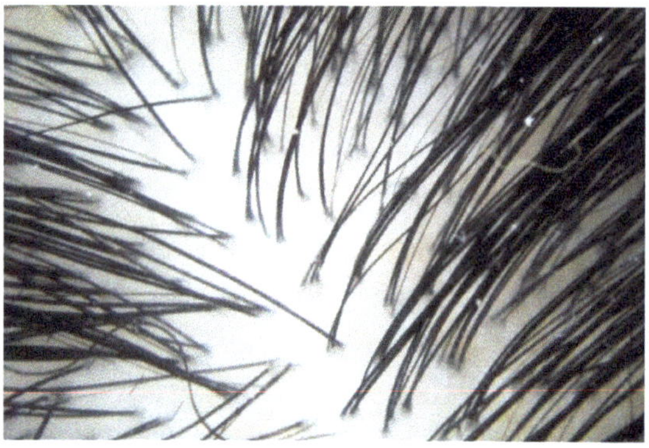

Figure 13.1 **Trichoscopy of traction alopecia (from Capilclinic.com, with permission).**

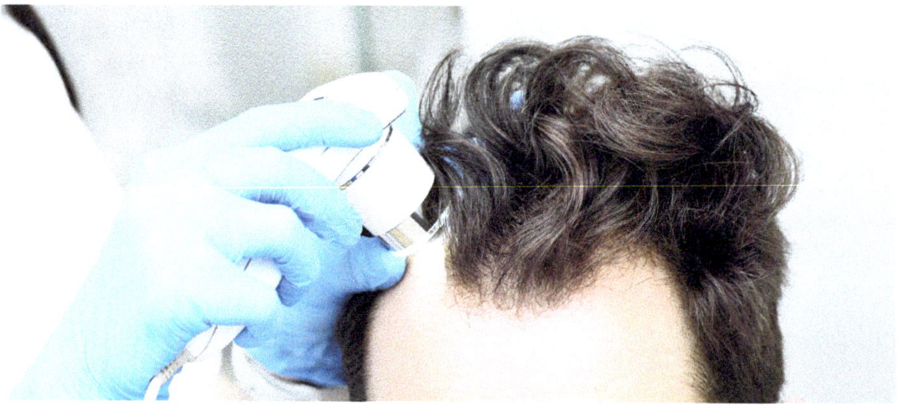

Figure 13.2 **Trichoscopy being performed on a patient (from Shutterstock, under license).**

(Figures 13.3 and 13.4), and the tissue sample is sent for histopathological examination. The biopsy results can provide definitive information about the type and extent of hair loss, as well as any underlying inflammatory or scarring processes.

By combining the insights gained from a thorough history taking and clinical examination, practitioners can develop a comprehensive understanding of each patient's unique hair loss presentation and identify the most appropriate diagnostic tests and treatment options.

Diagnostic Tools and Tests

In addition to clinical examination, various diagnostic tools and tests can be used to further evaluate patients with hair loss. These tools and tests can provide objective measures of hair density, shaft diameter, and growth rate, as well as assess the overall health and function of the scalp and hair follicles.

1. *Trichometry*: Trichometry refers to the quantitative assessment of hair density, diameter, and growth rate using specialized imaging devices. These devices, such as the TrichoScan or the FotoFinder, use high-resolution digital photography and image analysis software to provide

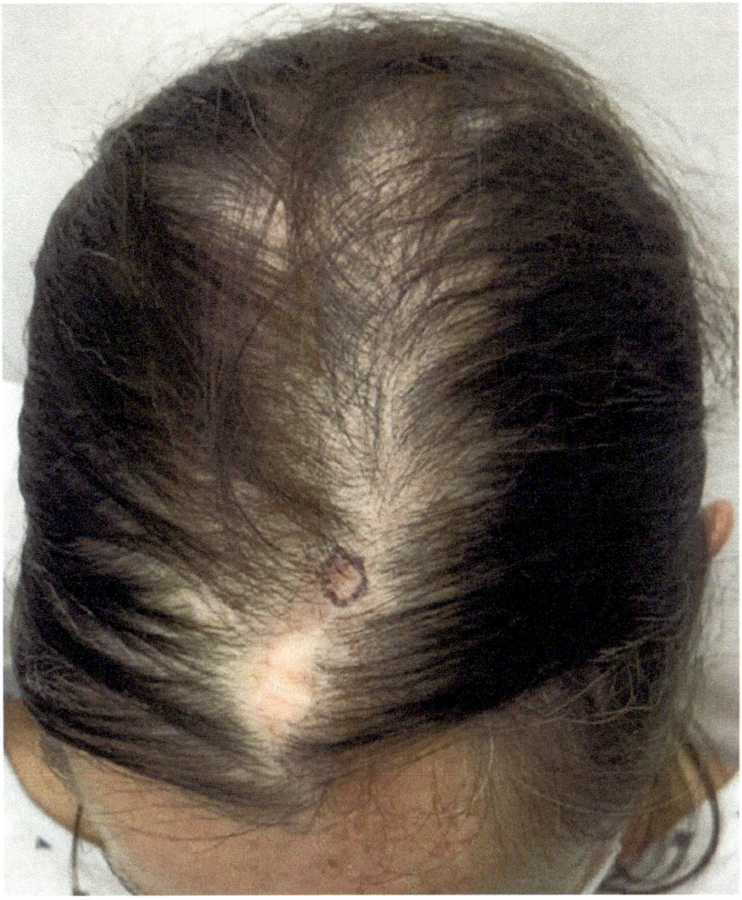

Figure 13.3 Biopsy site. (From AM Bailey, D Antonovich, Suture localization of scalp biopsy sites, *JAAD Online* 2022;87/1e1–e22, with permission).

objective measurements of hair parameters (Figures 13.5–13.7). It can be useful for monitoring treatment response over time and assessing the efficacy of non-surgical hair restoration interventions.

2. *Trichogram*: A trichogram is a microscopic examination of plucked hair fibers to assess the proportion of hairs in different stages of the hair growth cycle (anagen, catagen, and telogen). The test involves plucking a sample of hairs from the scalp and examining them under a microscope to determine the anagen-to-telogen ratio. An increased proportion of telogen hairs can indicate a diagnosis of telogen effluvium or other forms of hair cycle disruption.
3. *Phototrichogram*: A phototrichogram is a non-invasive method for assessing hair growth and shedding rates over time. The test involves shaving a small area of the scalp (typically 1–2 cm^2) and capturing serial photographs of the area at defined intervals (e.g., 2–3 days apart) (Figure 13.8). The photographs are then analyzed using image analysis software to determine the rate of hair growth and shedding. This can also be useful for monitoring treatment response and assessing the efficacy of hair growth promoters.
4. *Hair mineral analysis*: Hair mineral analysis is a test that measures the levels of various minerals and trace elements in a sample of hair. The test can provide insights into potential nutritional deficiencies or imbalances that may contribute to hair loss. However, the

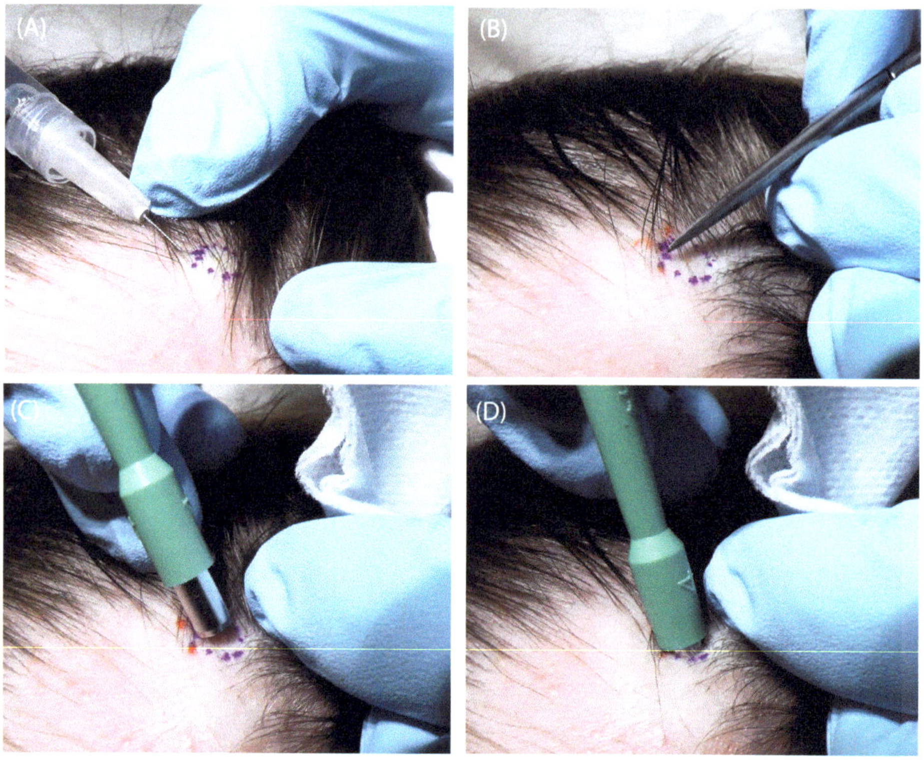

Figure 13.4 Punch biopsy site: (A) administration of anesthetic; (B) hairs are trimmed; (C) punch is angled parallel to the hair shaft; (D) rotate until the blade penetrates scalp. (From RS Haber, Scalp biopsy technique for the hair surgeon, *Hair Transplant Forum Int* 2013;23/5:162–4, with permission).

interpretation of hair mineral analysis results can be complex, and the test should be used in conjunction with other diagnostic tools and a thorough nutritional assessment.

5. *Hormonal testing*: In patients with suspected hormonal imbalances or conditions such as polycystic ovary syndrome (PCOS), hormonal testing may be indicated. This can include measurements of serum levels of androgens (e.g., testosterone, DHT), estrogens, and other relevant hormones (e.g., thyroid hormones, prolactin). Hormonal testing can help to identify underlying endocrine disorders that may contribute to hair loss and guide the selection of appropriate hormonal therapies.
6. *Genetic testing*: Genetic testing for hair loss is an emerging area of interest, particularly for patients with androgenetic alopecia. Several genetic polymorphisms, such as variations in the androgen receptor gene and the aromatase gene, have been associated with an increased risk of male and female-pattern hair loss. While genetic testing is not routinely used in clinical practice, it may be useful for identifying patients who are most likely to benefit from early intervention or for predicting response to certain treatments, such as finasteride.

By utilizing a combination of diagnostic tools and tests, practitioners can gain a more comprehensive understanding of each patient's hair loss condition and tailor their treatment approach accordingly. It is essential to interpret the results of these tests in the context of the patient's overall clinical presentation and to use them as an adjunct to, rather than a replacement for, thorough history taking and clinical examination.

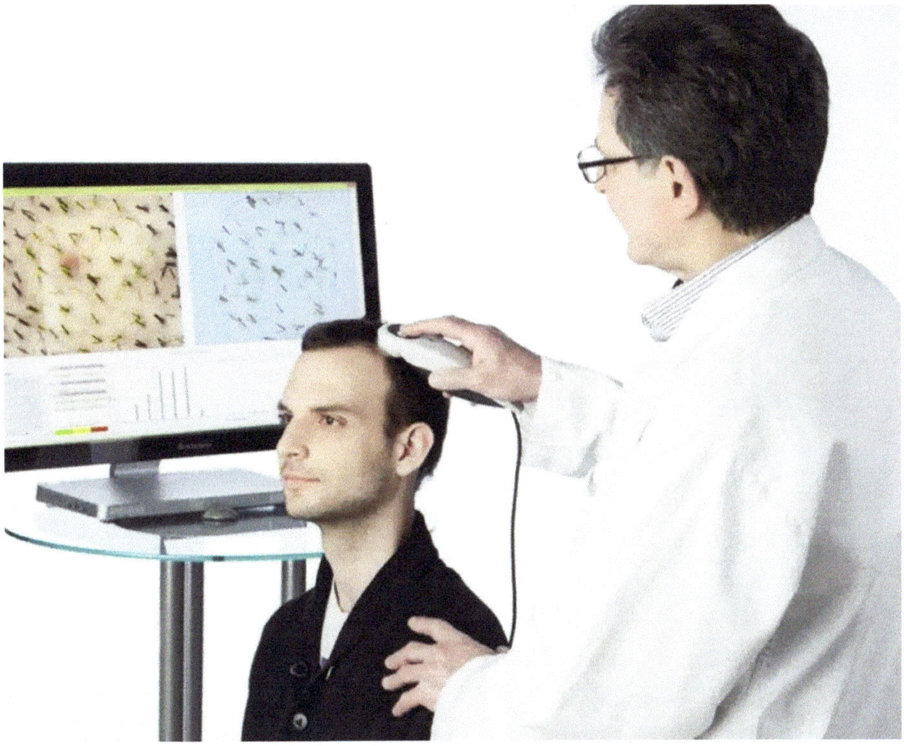

Figure 13.5 **A trichometry being performed (from www.vcaretrichology.com, with permission).**

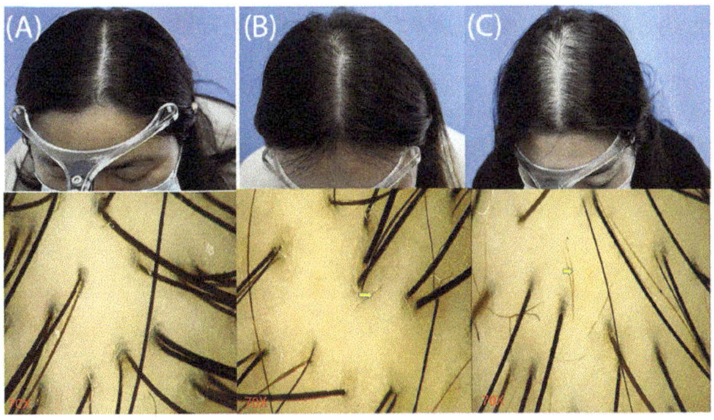

Figure 13.6 **Hair images taken by camera and TrichoScan at 70× magnification for female-pattern hair loss (FPHL) subjects and healthy controls. (A) Healthy controls; (B) subjects of Ludwig I; (C) subjects of Ludwig II. The yellow arrows show vellus hair (from Yang et al. 2022, with permission).**

Formulating a Treatment Plan

Once a comprehensive patient evaluation has been completed and a diagnosis has been established, the next step is to formulate a personalized treatment plan. This process involves considering the patient's specific hair loss presentation, medical history, and personal goals and preferences, as well as the available non-surgical hair restoration options and their potential risks and benefits.

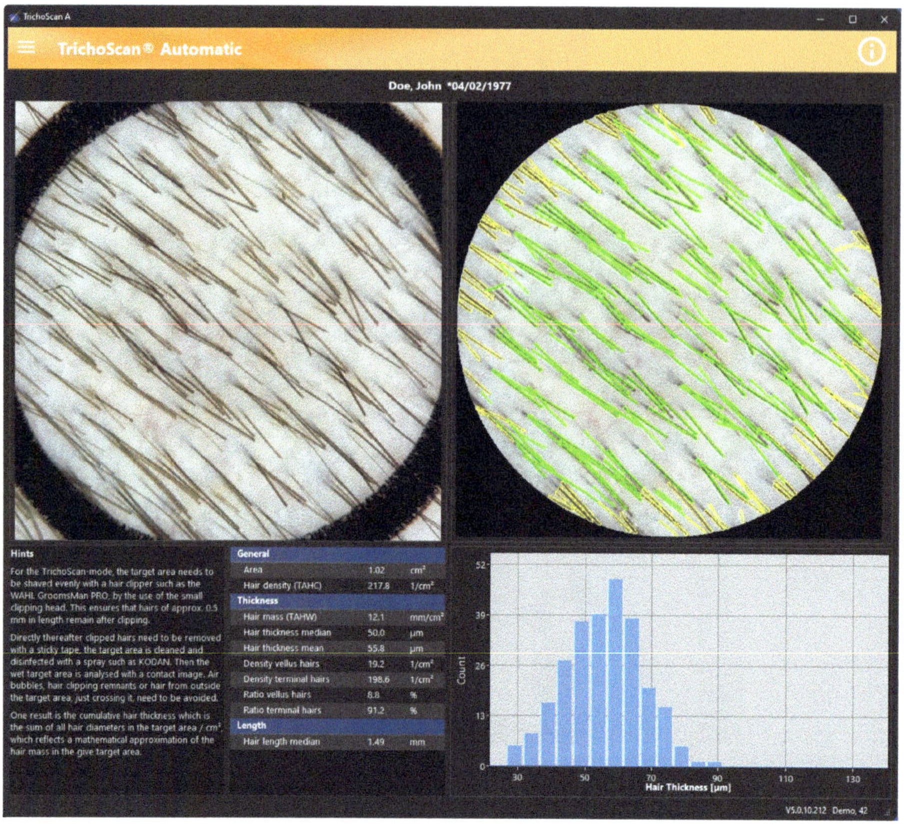

Figure 13.7 TrichoScan software interface (from www.Trichoscan.com, with permission).

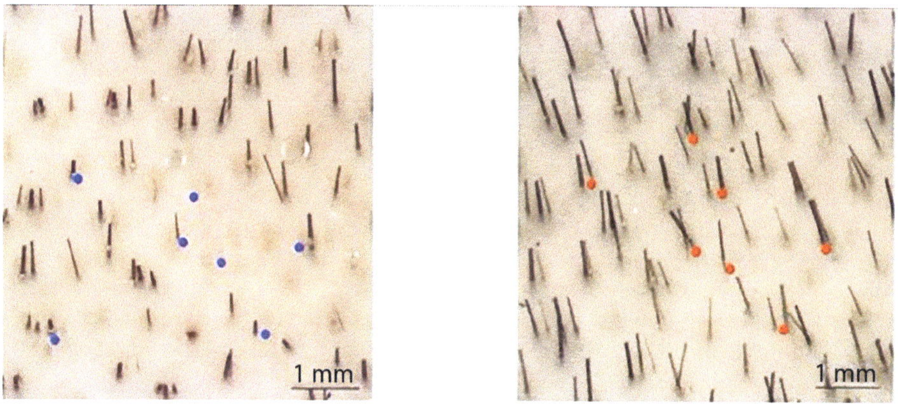

Figure 13.8 Phototrichogram evaluation before and after 4 months of treatment (from KeratinResearch.com, with permission).

Key considerations when formulating a treatment plan include:

1. *Type and extent of hair loss*: The type and extent of hair loss will largely determine the most appropriate treatment approach. For example, patients with early stage androgenetic alopecia may benefit from topical minoxidil or low-level laser therapy, while those with more advanced hair loss may require a combination of treatments, such as oral finasteride and platelet-rich plasma therapy.
2. *Patient age and gender*: The patient's age and gender can influence treatment selection, as certain interventions may be more effective or appropriate for specific age groups or genders. For example, oral finasteride is typically not recommended for women of childbearing age due to the risk of fetal abnormalities, while postmenopausal women may benefit from hormonal therapies such as spironolactone or topical estrogens.
3. *Medical history and comorbidities*: The patient's medical history and any coexisting conditions should be carefully considered when selecting hair loss treatments. Certain medical conditions, such as thyroid disorders or nutritional deficiencies, may need to be addressed concurrently to optimize treatment outcomes. Additionally, some hair loss treatments may be contraindicated in patients with specific medical conditions or those taking certain medications.
4. *Patient preferences and lifestyle*: The patient's personal preferences and lifestyle should be taken into account when formulating a treatment plan. Some patients may prefer non-invasive, topical treatments, while others may be willing to undergo more intensive interventions, such as platelet-rich plasma therapy or low-level laser therapy. It is essential to discuss the potential risks, benefits, and time commitments associated with each treatment option and to involve the patient in the decision-making process.
5. *Realistic expectations*: Setting realistic expectations is crucial for ensuring patient satisfaction and adherence to treatment. Patients should be informed that non-surgical hair restoration interventions typically require a long-term commitment and that results may take several months to become apparent. It is also important to emphasize that the goal of treatment is to slow or halt hair loss progression and promote hair regrowth, rather than to restore hair density to its original, pre-loss state.
6. *Combination therapies*: In many cases, a combination of non-surgical hair restoration treatments may be necessary to achieve optimal results. For example, patients with androgenetic alopecia may benefit from a combination of oral finasteride, topical minoxidil, and low-level laser therapy. When considering combination therapies, it is essential to assess the potential for synergistic or additive effects, as well as any possible interactions or contraindications.
7. *Long-term management*: Hair loss is often a chronic condition that requires ongoing management and monitoring. When formulating a treatment plan, practitioners should consider the long-term sustainability and practicality of the selected interventions. This may involve periodic follow-up visits to assess treatment response, adjust dosages or frequencies, and address any adverse effects or concerns.

Treatment Plan Examples

1. Early-stage androgenetic alopecia (male or female-pattern hair loss)
   - Protocol example:
     - Start with topical minoxidil 5%, applied twice daily to affected areas.

    - Consider low-level laser therapy (LLLT) using FDA-cleared devices for patients open to non-invasive approaches.
    - Monitor patient progress at 3 and 6 months to assess response and compliance.
2. Advanced androgenetic alopecia
   - Protocol example:
     - Combine oral finasteride (1 mg daily) for male patients with topical minoxidil 5%.
     - For female patients, especially postmenopausal, consider spironolactone (50–100 mg daily) or topical estrogens under careful monitoring.
     - Add platelet-rich plasma (PRP) therapy administered monthly for the first 3 months, then quarterly as maintenance.
     - Discuss possible integration of hair transplant referral for patients seeking surgical options.
3. Telogen effluvium
   - Protocol example:
     - Address underlying triggers (e.g., thyroid dysfunction or nutritional deficiencies like iron or vitamin D).
     - Initiate biotin supplementation (5000 mcg daily) alongside treatment of the root cause.
     - Educate patients on the transient nature of this condition and provide reassurance.
     - Reassess after 3–6 months to evaluate hair regrowth.
4. Alopecia areata
   - Protocol example:
     - Start with intralesional corticosteroids (e.g., triamcinolone acetonide 5–10 mg/mL) for localized patches.
     - For extensive involvement, consider systemic corticosteroids or newer options like Janus kinase (JAK) inhibitors if available.
     - Monitor for autoimmune comorbidities and address them as needed.
5. Postmenopausal hair thinning
   - Protocol example:
     - Consider hormonal options such as low-dose estradiol cream applied topically or spironolactone for androgen reduction.
     - Combine with LLLT or minoxidil to enhance efficacy.
     - Counsel patients on gradual results and importance of adherence.
6. Long-term maintenance plan
   - Schedule follow-ups every 6–12 months to:
     - Monitor treatment efficacy and adherence.
     - Adjust dosages or add new therapies based on patient response.
     - Address any side effects and provide continuous education.
7. Combination therapy protocols
   - Example: Male androgenetic alopecia: Oral finasteride + Topical minoxidil + LLLT.
   - Example: Female androgenetic alopecia: Spironolactone + Topical minoxidil + PRP therapy.

By carefully considering these factors and tailoring treatment plans to each patient's unique needs and goals, practitioners can optimize the effectiveness and acceptability of non-surgical hair restoration interventions. A well-formulated treatment plan should be evidence-based, patient-centered, and flexible enough to accommodate changes in the patient's hair loss presentation or treatment preferences over time.

Conclusion

Effective patient evaluation and diagnosis form the foundation of successful non-surgical hair restoration. By performing a thorough history and clinical examinations, utilizing advanced diagnostic tools, and creating tailored treatment plans, practitioners can provide patients with the most suitable interventions for their unique hair loss conditions. Personalized treatment plans, built on evidence-based interventions and aligned with the patient's goals and preferences, are essential to achieving optimal outcomes. Practitioners must also set realistic expectations, consider combination therapies, and incorporate long-term management to ensure sustained success and patient satisfaction. As advancements in hair restoration continue to emerge, practitioners who remain informed and adaptable will be best positioned to deliver exceptional care. By mastering patient evaluation and diagnosis, practitioners can build trust, achieve superior outcomes, and establish themselves as leaders in the field of non-surgical hair restoration. The following chapters will explore treatment protocols, patient management strategies, and practical considerations for creating a thriving hair restoration practice, offering a complete toolkit for providing exceptional care.

Chapter 14

Treatment Protocols and Guidelines

Julyssa A. Renteria and Robert Dorfman

Introduction

Establishing clear, evidence-based treatment protocols is key for delivering consistent, high-quality care in non-surgical hair restoration. These protocols provide practitioners with a structured approach to implementing interventions, monitoring patient progress, and making necessary adjustments to therapy. This chapter explores the development of individualized treatment plans, the rationale for combining therapies, and the importance of ongoing evaluation and refinement. By adhering to best practices, practitioners can optimize outcomes, minimize risks, and ensure the highest standard of care for their patients.

Developing Individualized Treatment Plans

The cornerstone of effective non-surgical hair restoration is the development of individualized treatment plans that are tailored to each patient's unique hair loss presentation, medical history, and personal goals. This process requires a thoughtful integration of insights from patient evaluation and diagnosis, combined with a comprehensive understanding of available treatment options, including their risks and benefits.

Key steps in developing individualized treatment plans include:

1. *Defining treatment goals*: The first step in creating a personalized treatment plan is to establish clear, realistic goals in collaboration with the patient. These goals may include slowing or halting hair loss progression, promoting hair regrowth, improving hair density and thickness, and enhancing overall scalp health. It is essential to ensure that the patient's expectations are aligned with the likely outcomes of the selected interventions and to emphasize the importance of long-term commitment and adherence to the treatment plan.

 DOI: 10.1201/9781032726397-14

2. *Selecting appropriate interventions*: Based on the patient's specific hair loss diagnosis, severity, and pattern, as well as their age, gender, and medical history, the practitioner should select the most appropriate non-surgical hair restoration interventions. This may involve a single therapy or a combination of treatments, such as topical minoxidil, low-level laser therapy, platelet-rich plasma therapy, or nutritional supplements. The choice of interventions should be evidence-based and take into account the patient's preferences, lifestyle, and any potential contraindications or interactions with existing medications.
3. *Determining treatment frequencies and durations*: Once the appropriate interventions have been selected, the practitioner should establish the optimal treatment frequencies and durations based on the available evidence and clinical experience. This may involve specifying the daily application of topical medications, the number and spacing of in-office treatments, or the duration of oral supplement regimens. It is important to provide patients with clear, written instructions on how to administer or undergo each intervention to ensure optimal compliance and treatment efficacy.
4. *Setting expectations and milestones*: To maintain patient motivation and adherence, it is crucial to set realistic expectations regarding the timeline for visible results and the extent of hair regrowth or improvement that can be achieved. Practitioners should establish clear milestones for assessing treatment response, such as follow-up appointments at 3, 6, and 12 months, and discuss the potential need for long-term maintenance therapy. I often liken the application of topical minoxidil or finasteride to brushing your teeth before bed—it's a simple routine that, once integrated, becomes a natural and essential part of daily life. Framing treatment this way can help patients view their regimen as a manageable, ongoing habit rather than a burden. This approach fosters a collaborative, transparent relationship between the practitioner and patient and promotes a shared understanding of the treatment journey.
5. *Incorporating patient education and support*: Effective individualized treatment plans should also include a strong emphasis on patient education and support. This may involve providing patients with written materials or online resources on the nature of their hair loss condition, the rationale behind the selected interventions, and the importance of adherence and long-term management. Practitioners should also offer ongoing support and guidance to help patients navigate any challenges or concerns that may arise during the treatment process, such as managing side effects or adjusting to new hair care routines.

By adopting a comprehensive, patient-centered approach to treatment planning, practitioners can ensure each patient receives tailored and effective non-surgical hair restoration therapies. This approach not only optimizes outcomes but also enhances patient satisfaction and long-term adherence to recommended treatments.

Combining Multiple Therapies for Optimal Results

In many cases, combining multiple non-surgical hair restoration therapies can lead to better outcomes compared to monotherapy. This synergistic approach leverages the distinct mechanisms of action and potential additive or complementary effects of different interventions, addressing hair loss from multiple angles and maximizing the overall treatment response.

The rationale for combining therapies includes:

1. *Targeting multiple pathways*: Hair loss is often a multifactorial process involving various underlying mechanisms, such as genetic predisposition, hormonal imbalances, nutrient deficiencies, and environmental stressors. By combining therapies that target different pathways, such as oral finasteride to address hormonal influences and low-level laser therapy to stimulate cellular metabolism, practitioners can provide a more comprehensive and effective treatment approach.
2. *Enhancing treatment efficacy*: Certain combinations of non-surgical hair restoration therapies have been shown to yield superior results compared to monotherapy in clinical studies. For example, the combination of topical minoxidil and oral finasteride has been found to produce greater improvements in hair count and density than either treatment alone in patients with androgenetic alopecia. Similarly, the addition of platelet-rich plasma therapy to topical minoxidil or low-level laser therapy has been associated with enhanced hair regrowth and patient satisfaction.
3. *Addressing individual variability*: Patients may exhibit variable responses to different hair loss interventions due to factors such as genetic variations, age, and the severity or duration of their condition. By combining multiple therapies, practitioners can increase the likelihood of achieving a satisfactory treatment response in a broader range of patients, as individuals who may not respond optimally to one intervention may benefit from the synergistic effects of another.
4. *Targeting different stages of the hair growth cycle*: The hair growth cycle, as discussed in previous chapters, consists of three main phases: anagen (growth), catagen (transition), and telogen (resting). Different non-surgical hair restoration therapies may exert their effects at various stages of this cycle. For example, topical minoxidil is believed to prolong the anagen phase and promote the transition of follicles from the telogen to the anagen phase, while low-level laser therapy may stimulate cellular metabolism and improve the overall health and function of the hair follicles.

Examples of evidence-based combinations for non-surgical hair restoration include:

- Topical minoxidil + Oral finasteride for androgenetic alopecia (Van Neste 2020)
- Low-level laser therapy + Topical minoxidil for androgenetic alopecia (Pillai and Mysore 2021)
- Platelet-rich plasma therapy + Topical minoxidil or low-level laser therapy for androgenetic alopecia (Alves and Grimalt 2018)
- Nutritional supplements (e.g., biotin, iron, vitamin D) + Topical minoxidil or oral finasteride for telogen effluvium or androgenetic alopecia

When combining therapies, I generally recommend that patients use both minoxidil and a 5-alpha reductase inhibitor (such as finasteride or dutasteride). Whether they choose topical or oral formulations depends on what they find easiest to incorporate into their routine. Ideally, both medications should be included, as this combination tends to yield the best results. However, some male patients express concerns about the potential sexual side effects associated with finasteride or dutasteride. For these patients, I emphasize the importance of at least using minoxidil, though combining both is preferable.

In addition, I recommend incorporating a hair vitamin containing nutrients like biotin, vitamin D, zinc, and iron, as well as low-level laser therapy for at-home use. For in-office treatments, options such as platelet-rich plasma, exosome therapy, or a 1927 nm thulium laser session can enhance outcomes. Ideally, patients could utilize all these treatments; however, it's essential to have a thoughtful discussion about their budget, preferences, and lifestyle. This ensures the treatment plan is not only effective but also practical and tailored to the individual's needs. A personalized, realistic regimen increases the likelihood of adherence and long-term success.

Practitioners must consider potential interactions, contraindications, and adverse effects when combining multiple therapies. Reviewing evidence on the safety and efficacy of specific combinations and closely monitoring patients for signs of intolerance or unexpected reactions is essential. Regular monitoring and adjustment of treatment plans are vital for successful non-surgical hair restoration. Follow-up appointments enable practitioners to evaluate treatment response, address adverse effects or compliance issues, and modify interventions as necessary to achieve the best results.

Key considerations for monitoring and adjusting treatment plans include:

1. *Assessing treatment response*: Practitioners should establish a standardized protocol for evaluating treatment response at regular intervals, such as 3, 6, and 12 months after initiating therapy. This may involve a combination of subjective assessments, such as patient-reported improvements in hair density, thickness, or shedding, and objective measures, such as serial photography, trichoscopy, or hair counts. By tracking treatment response over time, practitioners can determine the effectiveness of the prescribed interventions and make informed decisions about whether to continue, modify, or discontinue specific therapies.
2. *Monitoring for adverse effects*: Non-surgical hair restoration therapies, while generally well-tolerated, can be associated with certain adverse effects, such as scalp irritation, itching, or unwanted hair growth in non-target areas. During follow-up appointments, practitioners should inquire about any side effects or tolerability issues experienced by the patient and perform a thorough scalp examination to identify any signs of irritation, inflammation, or other complications. If significant adverse effects are noted, the practitioner may need to adjust the prescribed regimen, such as reducing the frequency or concentration of a topical medication or temporarily suspending a particular therapy.
3. *Assessing patient compliance and satisfaction*: Treatment adherence is a critical factor in the success of non-surgical hair restoration interventions. During follow-up visits, practitioners should assess patient compliance with the prescribed regimen, inquiring about any challenges or barriers to adherence and providing support and guidance as needed. It is also important to gauge patient satisfaction with the treatment process and outcomes, as this can impact long-term adherence and the overall patient–practitioner relationship. If compliance or satisfaction issues are identified, the practitioner may need to provide additional education, modify the treatment plan to better align with the patient's preferences or lifestyle, or explore alternative interventions.
4. *Adjusting treatment plans based on response and evolving needs*: As patients progress through their non-surgical hair restoration journey, their treatment needs and goals may evolve. For example, a patient who initially presents with mild androgenetic alopecia and responds well to topical minoxidil may require the addition of oral finasteride or low-level laser therapy as their condition progresses over time. Alternatively, a patient who experiences a plateau in treatment response after several months of therapy may benefit from the addition of

platelet-rich plasma therapy or a change in the prescribed regimen. By continually reassessing treatment response and the patient's evolving needs, practitioners can ensure that the treatment plan remains optimized and effective over the long term.

5. *Documenting treatment adjustments and rationale*: Whenever modifications are made to a patient's non-surgical hair restoration treatment plan, it is essential to document the changes and the rationale behind them in the patient's medical record. This documentation should include details on the specific interventions added, discontinued, or modified, as well as the reasons for the adjustments, such as changes in treatment response, adverse effects, or patient preferences. Clear and comprehensive documentation not only promotes continuity of care but also serves as a valuable reference for future treatment decisions and communication with other healthcare providers.

Conclusion

Establishing clear, evidence-based treatment plans is key to delivering effective and consistent care in non-surgical hair restoration. By integrating comprehensive patient evaluations with tailored treatment plans, practitioners can address individual needs and optimize outcomes. Strategic use of combination therapies, when supported by evidence, offers a nuanced approach to tackling hair loss, leveraging synergistic effects to enhance efficacy and patient satisfaction. Ongoing monitoring ensures treatment plans remain dynamic and responsive, allowing practitioners to refine interventions as needed to accommodate changes in patient progress and preferences. This iterative approach not only improves clinical outcomes but also reinforces patient trust and engagement. As advancements in non-surgical hair restoration evolve, staying informed of emerging research and techniques will empower practitioners to provide innovative, patient-centered care. Looking ahead, the following chapters will focus on managing patient expectations, strengthening communication, and scaling a successful practice, equipping practitioners to excel in a rapidly evolving field and deliver transformative results for their patients.

Chapter 15

Managing Patient Expectations

Julyssa A. Renteria and Robert Dorfman

Introduction

Managing patient expectations is essential for delivering high-quality, patient-centered care in non-surgical hair restoration. Patients often approach treatment with high hopes for transformative outcomes, and it is the practitioner's role to align these expectations with achievable, evidence-based results. This chapter delves into strategies for effective communication, goal setting, and addressing common misconceptions about non-surgical hair restoration. By fostering clear, open dialogue and setting realistic, attainable objectives, practitioners can build trust, promote adherence to treatment plans, and ultimately enhance both patient satisfaction and clinical outcomes.

Communicating Effectively with Patients

Effective communication is the foundation of successful patient expectation management in non-surgical hair restoration. By establishing clear, open, and empathetic communication with patients from the initial consultation and throughout the treatment journey, practitioners can build trust, rapport, and a shared understanding of the goals, limitations, and potential outcomes of the prescribed interventions. Key strategies for communicating effectively with patients are described in the following.

Practitioners should prioritize active listening during patient consultations, focusing fully on the patient's concerns, questions, and expectations. This involves not only hearing the patient's words but also understanding the emotions, motivations, and values that underpin their concerns about hair loss and treatment goals. Demonstrating genuine interest and empathy fosters a safe and supportive environment, encouraging patients to share openly and honestly.

When discussing hair loss diagnosis, treatment options, and expected outcomes, practitioners should communicate in clear and straightforward language. Avoiding technical jargon and using relatable analogies, visual aids, or patient-friendly materials can help convey complex information effectively. Providing patients ample opportunity to ask questions or clarify uncertainties ensures they fully understand their condition and the proposed treatment plan, promoting informed decision-making.

DOI: 10.1201/9781032726397-15

Setting realistic expectations is a cornerstone of effective patient management. Practitioners should be transparent about the limitations of current therapies, the variability in individual responses, and the likely outcomes based on the patient's unique circumstances. Honest discussions from the beginning helps patients avoid frustration or disappointment, fostering trust and collaboration in the treatment process.

Hair loss can have a profound emotional impact, making it important for practitioners to approach these conversations with empathy and validation. Acknowledging the patient's feelings and normalizing their concerns reassures them that their experiences are understood and respected. Offering compassionate support throughout the treatment process empowers patients and helps build a trusting patient–provider relationship.

Effective communication must be tailored to each patient's unique needs and preferences. Some patients may appreciate detailed scientific explanations, while others may prefer relatable, emotional language. By adapting their communication style to the individual, practitioners can ensure that information is delivered in a way that resonates, facilitating understanding and engagement.

Communication should extend beyond the initial consultation and be maintained throughout the treatment journey. Regular follow-up appointments provide opportunities to assess treatment progress, address concerns or side effects, and offer continued guidance and support. Practitioners can also check in between appointments to share updates, offer encouragement, or provide additional resources. Consistent, ongoing communication fosters a strong practitioner–patient relationship and ensures patients feel supported and informed at every stage of their hair restoration journey (Ali and Feldman 2014; Poulos et al. 2008; Chang et al. 2022; Ubbink et al. 2016).

Setting Realistic Goals

Setting realistic goals is another component of managing patient expectations in non-surgical hair restoration. By working collaboratively with patients to establish clear, achievable objectives for their treatment, practitioners can help ensure that patients have an accurate understanding of what can be accomplished with the prescribed interventions and avoid disappointment or frustration down the line.

Key considerations for setting realistic goals include:

1. *Assessing patient expectations*: During the initial consultation, practitioners should carefully assess the patient's expectations for their hair restoration treatment. This may involve asking open-ended questions about their desired outcomes, such as "What are you hoping to achieve with this treatment?" or "How do you envision your hair looking after the intervention?" By gaining a clear understanding of the patient's hopes and expectations, practitioners can identify any unrealistic or misaligned goals and work to adjust them based on the available evidence and the patient's unique characteristics. For example, a patient might express a desire to achieve the same hair density they had in their early 20s, despite presenting with advanced androgenetic alopecia and significant follicular miniaturization. In such a case, the practitioner could respond by saying:

   > "I understand that restoring your hair to its original density is something you're hoping for, and I appreciate you sharing that goal with me. While our current treatments are effective at slowing hair loss and promoting some regrowth, achieving that level

of density may not be possible. However, we can focus on strengthening your existing hair, improving its thickness, and optimizing overall scalp health to create a noticeable improvement in volume and appearance. Let's work together to set a realistic plan to achieve the best possible results for you."

This approach balances empathy with honesty, helping the patient set realistic expectations while maintaining their trust and confidence in the treatment plan. Despite the practitioner's best efforts to set realistic goals, some patients may still harbor unrealistic expectations about the potential outcomes of their hair restoration treatment. In these cases, practitioners should address these expectations directly and compassionately, using evidence-based information and patient education to help realign the patient's goals with what is achievable. This may involve having difficult but necessary conversations about the limitations of current therapies or the potential need for adjunctive treatments, such as surgical hair restoration, in cases of advanced or refractory hair loss.

2. *Providing evidence-based information*: When discussing potential treatment outcomes, practitioners should provide patients with accurate, evidence-based information about the efficacy and limitations of the proposed interventions. This may involve sharing clinical trial data, before-and-after photos of similar cases, or patient testimonials that demonstrate realistic results. By grounding the conversation in objective, scientific evidence, practitioners can help patients develop a more accurate understanding of what can be achieved with non-surgical hair restoration therapies.
3. *Explaining individual variability*: It is essential for practitioners to emphasize the individual variability of treatment responses in non-surgical hair restoration. Patients should be made aware that factors such as age, gender, genetic predisposition, and the severity and duration of their hair loss can all impact the effectiveness of the prescribed interventions. By acknowledging the unique nature of each patient's hair restoration journey, practitioners can help manage expectations and avoid comparisons to unrealistic or unrepresentative cases.
4. *Discussing timeline and maintenance*: When setting treatment goals, practitioners should also discuss the expected timeline for visible results and the importance of long-term maintenance. Patients should be informed that non-surgical hair restoration interventions typically require several months of consistent use before significant improvements are seen and that ongoing treatment may be necessary to maintain the achieved results. By setting realistic expectations about the time course and long-term commitment required for successful hair restoration, practitioners can help patients develop a more patient, committed mindset. As discussed in previous chapters, it is important to create measurable milestones to track treatment progress.

By taking a proactive, evidence-based approach to setting realistic goals, practitioners can help patients develop a clear, accurate understanding of what can be achieved with non-surgical hair restoration interventions. This not only helps to manage expectations and avoid disappointment but also fosters a more positive, collaborative treatment experience that ultimately leads to improved patient satisfaction and outcomes.

Addressing Concerns and Complications

Even with the most effective communication and goal-setting strategies, patients undergoing non-surgical hair restoration may still experience concerns, complications, or dissatisfaction with their treatment progress. Practitioners should be prepared to address these issues promptly, compassionately, and effectively to maintain patient trust and engagement and optimize long-term outcomes. Common concerns and complications that may arise during non-surgical hair restoration treatment are discussed next.

While non-surgical hair restoration interventions are generally well-tolerated, some patients may experience side effects or discomfort related to their treatment. These may include scalp irritation, redness, itching, or flaking with topical minoxidil; sexual side effects or gynecomastia with oral finasteride; or pain, swelling, or bruising with platelet-rich plasma injections. When patients report these issues, practitioners should take them seriously, assess their severity and impact, and work collaboratively with the patient to develop a plan for managing or mitigating the side effects. This may involve adjusting the dose or frequency of the prescribed intervention, recommending adjunctive therapies or lifestyle modifications to improve tolerability, or, in rare cases, discontinuing the treatment altogether.

Some patients may experience slower or less robust hair regrowth than expected based on the available evidence or the practitioner's initial projections. In these cases, it is essential for practitioners to remain empathetic, supportive, and proactive in addressing the patient's concerns. This may involve reassessing the patient's diagnosis and treatment plan, considering the addition of adjunctive therapies or lifestyle modifications to optimize results, or adjusting the patient's expectations based on their individual response. Practitioners should also emphasize the importance of patience and persistence in the hair restoration journey, reminding patients that visible improvements may take several months to manifest and that consistent, long-term adherence to the prescribed regimen is critical for success.

Non-surgical hair restoration interventions often require a significant level of patient commitment and adherence to achieve optimal results. Some patients may struggle with consistency, forget to use their prescribed products, or become discouraged by the slow pace of progress. In these cases, practitioners should work to identify the underlying barriers to adherence and develop strategies to support and motivate the patient. This may involve engaging in motivational interviewing, providing additional education on the importance of consistent use, offering reminder systems or adherence aids, or exploring alternative treatment options that better fit the patient's lifestyle and preferences. Practitioners should also emphasize the long-term benefits of adherence and the potential consequences of inconsistent or interrupted treatment, such as the loss of achieved hair regrowth or the acceleration of further hair loss.

Despite the provider's best efforts to set realistic expectations and optimize treatment response, some patients may still express dissatisfaction with their hair restoration outcomes. In these cases, it is essential for practitioners to validate the patient's concerns, acknowledge the limitations of current therapies, and work collaboratively to develop a plan for moving forward. This may involve reassessing the patient's diagnosis and treatment plan, considering alternative or adjunctive interventions, or referring the patient to a hair restoration specialist for further evaluation or management. Providers should also emphasize the importance of open, honest communication and the value of the patient–provider relationship in navigating these challenges and finding a satisfactory resolution. This approach not only helps to optimize individual patient results but also strengthens the practitioner's reputation as a knowledgeable, compassionate, and effective provider in the field of hair restoration.

Examples of Managing Treatment Concerns

Managing Side Effects of Topical Minoxidil

- Concern: A patient using topical minoxidil reports scalp irritation, redness, and itching.
- Approach: Acknowledge the concern: "I understand how uncomfortable this irritation can be." Assess the severity and underlying cause. For mild cases, suggest switching to a foam formulation, which may have fewer irritants than the liquid form. Recommend supportive care, such as a gentle, fragrance-free shampoo to soothe the scalp. If symptoms persist, consider lowering the frequency of application or discontinuing the treatment temporarily while exploring alternatives, such as low-level laser therapy (LLLT).

Addressing Slow or Suboptimal Results

- Concern: A patient expresses frustration after 3 months of treatment, stating they see no visible improvement.
- Approach: Reassure the patient: "It's normal for hair restoration treatments to take several months to show noticeable results." Reevaluate the treatment plan to ensure it aligns with their specific hair loss condition. If appropriate, consider adding adjunctive therapies, such as platelet-rich plasma (PRP) or low-dose oral minoxidil, to enhance outcomes. Reinforce the importance of adherence and consistency, reminding the patient that significant improvements often require at least 6–12 months of sustained effort.

Managing Fear of Systemic Side Effects

- Concern: A male patient using oral finasteride expresses anxiety about the potential for sexual side effects.
- Approach: Provide evidence-based information: "Clinical studies show that these side effects are rare and reversible upon discontinuation of the medication." Offer alternatives, such as topical finasteride, which has lower systemic absorption and a reduced risk of such effects. Monitor closely with regular follow-ups and encourage the patient to report any concerns immediately.

Overcoming Adherence Challenges

- Concern: A patient admits they often forget to apply their topical treatment or attend follow-up appointments.
- Approach: Explore the underlying reasons for non-adherence, such as inconvenience or forgetfulness. Suggest practical solutions, such as setting reminders on their phone or incorporating treatment into their daily routine. Offer simpler or more manageable alternatives, like combining treatments (e.g., topical finasteride and minoxidil) into a single application if available.

Addressing Unrealistic Expectations

- Concern: A patient with advanced androgenetic alopecia expresses disappointment that their hair density hasn't returned to its youthful state after 6 months of treatment.

- Approach: Gently reset expectations: "I understand your desire for a full restoration, but with the severity of your condition, our goal is to improve density and slow further loss rather than recreate the exact hairline you had in your 20s." Highlight achieved progress, such as improved thickness or scalp coverage. Discuss options for enhancing results, such as combining therapies or considering surgical hair restoration for denser regrowth.

Managing Emotional Distress

- Concern: A patient expresses emotional distress and low confidence due to their hair loss, despite treatment progress.
- Approach: Validate their feelings: "It's completely understandable to feel this way; hair loss can impact self-esteem." Offer additional support, such as referrals to counseling or support groups, if needed. Reinforce the positive aspects of their treatment journey and discuss realistic next steps to continue improving their outcomes.

Conclusion

Managing patient expectations is essential for delivering effective, patient-centered care in non-surgical hair restoration. Clear communication, realistic goal-setting, and proactive solutions to challenges build trust and foster adherence, ultimately enhancing patient satisfaction and outcomes. By combining empathy with evidence-based guidance, practitioners can align a patient's hopes with achievable results and navigate challenges such as side effects or adherence issues effectively. As the field evolves, staying informed and patient-focused ensures the highest quality care and successful treatment outcomes. The next chapters will explore building a thriving practice, ethical considerations, and emerging innovations in hair restoration.

Chapter 16

Building and Expanding a Hair Restoration Practice

Julyssa A. Renteria and Robert Dorfman

Introduction

Building and expanding a successful hair restoration practice requires a combination of clinical expertise, business acumen, and patient-centered care. As the demand for non-surgical hair restoration treatments continues to grow, practitioners who can effectively navigate the challenges and opportunities of this dynamic field will be well-positioned to thrive and make a meaningful impact in the lives of their patients. This chapter explores the key strategies and considerations for establishing and growing a hair restoration practice, including setting up a practice, marketing and attracting patients, and expanding the practice's space and services. By implementing these strategies and continually adapting to the evolving landscape of hair restoration, practitioners can build a thriving, rewarding practice that delivers exceptional care and outcomes to patients.

Setting Up a Practice

Establishing a successful hair restoration practice begins with careful planning, execution, and attention to detail. Key steps in setting up a practice include:

1. *Defining the practice's mission, values, and unique value proposition*: Practitioners should clearly articulate the core mission and values of their hair restoration practice, as well as the unique factors that set them apart from competitors. This may include specialized expertise, innovative treatment approaches, a commitment to patient education and empowerment, or a focus on delivering personalized, compassionate care.
   - Mission statement
     - *Example*: "Our mission is to empower individuals experiencing hair loss by providing personalized, evidence-based, and compassionate care that restores not only hair but also confidence and quality of life."

DOI: 10.1201/9781032726397-16

- Core values
  - *Example*: A practice may prioritize transparency, patient education, and innovation, highlighting these values by offering detailed consultations, providing accessible educational resources, and consistently adopting the latest non-surgical technologies.
- Unique value proposition
  - *Example*: A practitioner specializing in women's hair loss might emphasize expertise in treating conditions such as postpartum hair loss or hair thinning related to polycystic ovary syndrome. Alternatively, a practice with cutting-edge technology, like advanced trichoscopy imaging or personalized genomic testing, could position itself as the go-to destination for precision hair restoration.
- Commitment to patient empowerment
  - *Example*: Offering workshops or webinars on understanding hair loss conditions and treatments demonstrates a commitment to patient education. For instance, a practice might host monthly "Hair Health 101" sessions to answer questions and build trust with potential and current patients.
- Compassionate, personalized care
  - *Example*: A practice that follows up with patients after each session, offers custom-tailored treatment plans, and dedicates time to address emotional aspects of hair loss underscores its commitment to creating a supportive and empathetic environment.

By defining and showcasing their mission, values, and unique strengths through real-world examples, practitioners can build a compelling identity that resonates with patients and sets the stage for long-term success.

2. *Choosing an appropriate location and space*: The location and physical space of a hair restoration practice can have a significant impact on patient experience, operational efficiency, and overall success. Practitioners should carefully consider factors such as accessibility, parking, visibility, and competition when selecting a location. The practice space should be designed to create a welcoming, comfortable, and professional environment that reflects the practice's mission and values. This may include investing in high-quality furnishings, lighting, and decor that promote relaxation and confidence.
3. *Investing in essential equipment and technology*: Non-surgical hair restoration treatments often require specialized equipment and technology, such as low-level laser therapy devices, lasers, platelet-rich plasma preparation systems, medical-grade freezers for storage, and high-resolution imaging tools that have been discussed in previous chapters. Practitioners should carefully research and invest in reliable, evidence-based equipment that aligns with their treatment offerings and budget. This may involve partnering with reputable vendors, attending industry conferences and workshops, and seeking guidance from experienced colleagues.
4. *Building a skilled, patient-centered team*: A successful hair restoration practice relies on a skilled, compassionate, and collaborative team of professionals. Practitioners should prioritize hiring and training staff members who share their commitment to exceptional patient care, ongoing learning, and ethical practice. This may include medical assistants, nurses, physician assistants, patient coordinators, and administrative personnel who can support the practitioner in delivering seamless, personalized care to every patient.
5. *Developing efficient operational systems and protocols*: Streamlined, efficient operational systems are essential for managing patient flow, treatment delivery, and overall practice productivity. Practitioners should invest time and resources in developing clear, standardized protocols for patient intake, assessment, treatment planning, and follow-up care. This may involve implementing electronic health record systems, appointment scheduling software, and inventory management tools that optimize practice efficiency and minimize errors.

By carefully addressing these key elements of practice setup, hair restoration practitioners can create a strong, patient-centered foundation for long-term success and growth.

Marketing and Attracting Patients

Effective marketing and patient attraction strategies are critical for building a thriving hair restoration practice.

Key considerations for marketing and attracting patients include:

1. *Defining the target patient population*: Practitioners should have a clear understanding of their ideal patient population, including demographic characteristics, hair loss concerns, and treatment preferences. This may involve conducting market research, analyzing patient feedback and outcomes data, and staying abreast of industry trends and best practices. By tailoring marketing and outreach efforts to the specific needs and preferences of their target audience, practitioners can more effectively attract and retain patients who are likely to benefit from their services.
2. *Developing a strong online presence*: In today's digital age, a strong online presence is essential for attracting and engaging prospective patients. Practitioners should invest in a professional, user-friendly website that clearly communicates their expertise, services, and unique value proposition. The website should feature engaging, informative content that educates patients about hair loss causes, treatment options, and the practice's approach to care. Practitioners should also prioritize search engine optimization (SEO) strategies to improve their website's visibility and rankings for relevant keywords.
3. *Leveraging social media and digital marketing*: Social media platforms, such as Facebook, Instagram, and Twitter, offer powerful tools for connecting with prospective patients, sharing educational content, and showcasing patient success stories (Shauly et al. 2023; Bank et al. 2023). Practitioners should develop a consistent, engaging social media presence that aligns with their practice's mission and values. This may involve regularly posting informative articles, before-and-after photos, and patient testimonials that demonstrate the practice's expertise and commitment to exceptional care. Targeted digital advertising campaigns, such as Google AdWords and Facebook Ads, can also be effective for reaching specific patient populations and driving website traffic.
4. *Building referral networks and partnerships*: Referral networks and partnerships with other healthcare providers, such as dermatologists, endocrinologists, and primary care physicians, can be valuable sources of patient referrals and collaborative care opportunities. Practitioners should actively seek out and nurture relationships with referring providers who share their commitment to evidence-based, patient-centered care. This may involve hosting educational events, providing informational materials, and establishing clear communication channels for coordinating patient care.
5. *Offering educational events and resources*: Educational events and resources, such as seminars, webinars, and e-books, can be effective for attracting prospective patients and establishing the practice as a trusted authority in hair restoration. Practitioners should develop engaging, informative content that addresses common patient concerns, treatment options, and the latest research and innovations in the field. These events and resources can be promoted through the practice's website, social media channels, and email marketing campaigns to reach a wider audience and generate patient interest.

By implementing a comprehensive, multifaceted marketing and patient attraction strategy, hair restoration practitioners can effectively reach and engage their target patient population, build trust and credibility, and ultimately grow their practice.

Expanding Practice Space and Services

As a hair restoration practice grows and evolves, practitioners may need to consider expanding their physical space and treatment offerings to meet the changing needs and preferences of their patient population. Key strategies for expanding practice space and services include:

1. *Assessing patient demand and market trends*: Before expanding practice space or services, practitioners should carefully assess patient demand and market trends to ensure that the proposed changes align with the needs and preferences of their target audience. This may involve analyzing patient feedback and outcomes data, conducting market research, and staying abreast of industry trends and best practices. By making data-driven decisions about expansion, practitioners can minimize risk and maximize the potential for long-term success.
2. *Developing a comprehensive business plan*: Expanding practice space or services requires careful planning and execution to ensure a smooth, successful transition. Practitioners should develop a comprehensive business plan that outlines the goals, strategies, and financial projections for the proposed expansion. This may include identifying potential locations or spaces for expansion, evaluating equipment and technology needs, and forecasting revenue and expenses. The business plan should also address staffing requirements, marketing strategies, and potential challenges or risks associated with the expansion.
3. *Investing in advanced training and certification*: Expanding treatment offerings may require practitioners to invest in advanced training and certification to ensure that they have the necessary skills and expertise to deliver safe, effective care. This may involve attending workshops, conferences, or fellowship programs focused on specific non-surgical hair restoration techniques. By continually investing in their own education and professional development, practitioners can stay at the forefront of the field and provide the highest quality care to their patients. Popular meetings and conferences include the Anti-Aging Medicine World Congress, held annually in Miami and Monaco. Other meetings include Vegas Cosmetic Surgery and The Aesthetic Show, both of which are held annually in Las Vegas.
4. *Partnering with industry leaders and innovators*: Collaborating with industry leaders and innovators can be a valuable strategy for expanding practice services and staying ahead of the curve in non-surgical hair restoration. Practitioners may consider partnering with companies that develop cutting-edge hair restoration technologies, such as new laser devices or regenerative medicine products, to offer exclusive or early access to these treatments for their patients. These partnerships can also provide opportunities for research collaboration, co-marketing initiatives, and professional networking that can help to grow and differentiate the practice.
5. *Emphasizing patient education and empowerment*: As a practice expands its space and services, it is essential to maintain a strong focus on patient education and empowerment. Practitioners should prioritize developing clear, informative materials that help patients understand the benefits, risks, and limitations of new treatment options, as well as the importance of realistic expectations and long-term maintenance. By empowering patients to

make informed decisions about their care and actively participate in their treatment journey, practitioners can build trust, loyalty, and satisfaction that will support the long-term success of the expanded practice.

Expanding practice space and services can be a complex, challenging process, but with careful planning, execution, and a commitment to patient-centered care, hair restoration practitioners can successfully navigate this growth phase and position their practice for long-term success.

Conclusion

Building and expanding a successful hair restoration practice requires a strategic blend of clinical expertise, business strategy, and a patient-centered approach. By defining a clear mission and values, investing in essential resources, and assembling a skilled team, practitioners can create a strong foundation for success. Effective marketing strategies, including defining target audiences, leveraging online platforms, and cultivating referral networks, are essential to attract and retain patients. As practices grow, assessing patient demand, planning thoughtfully, and embracing innovation through partnerships and advanced training ensure sustainable expansion. Ultimately, adaptability, innovation, and a focus on patient satisfaction are the cornerstones of success. By consistently delivering high-quality, personalized care, practitioners can establish themselves as leaders in the field and positively impact the lives of individuals experiencing hair loss. Future chapters will address legal and ethical considerations and explore emerging trends, equipping practitioners with the tools to navigate this evolving field with confidence and excellence.

Chapter 17

Legal and Ethical Considerations

Julyssa A. Renteria, Robert Dorfman and Robert Greer

Introduction

Non-surgical hair restoration, like any medical practice, is subject to a complex array of legal and ethical considerations that practitioners must navigate to ensure the safety, well-being, and trust of their patients. From regulatory compliance and informed consent to patient privacy and professional integrity, hair restoration practitioners must uphold the highest standards of legal and ethical conduct in every aspect of their practice. This chapter explores the key legal and ethical issues surrounding non-surgical hair restoration, providing guidance and best practices for practitioners to maintain compliance, mitigate risk, and prioritize patient welfare. By understanding and adhering to these critical principles, practitioners can build a practice that is not only successful but also ethical, responsible, and deserving of patient trust.

Regulatory Guidelines

Non-surgical hair restoration is subject to various regulatory guidelines at the federal, state, and local levels. The US Food and Drug Administration (FDA) regulates the safety and efficacy of drugs, devices, and biologics used in non-surgical hair restoration. Practitioners must ensure that any products they use, such as minoxidil, finasteride, or platelet-rich plasma preparation systems, are FDA approved for their intended use and that they follow all labeling, storage, and administration requirements. Off-label use of products, while common in medical practice, should be based on sound scientific evidence and accompanied by appropriate patient informed consent. Hair restoration practitioners must hold valid medical licenses in the states where they practice and adhere to the defined scope of practice for their specialty. This may include specific requirements for training, certification, and continuing education in non-surgical hair restoration techniques. Practitioners should also be aware of any state-specific regulations or restrictions on the use of certain treatments or technologies, such as laser devices or regenerative medicine products. Practitioners must ensure that their advertising and marketing practices comply with federal and state regulations, such as the Federal Trade Commission's (FTC) truth-in-advertising rules. This

DOI: 10.1201/9781032726397-17

includes avoiding false, misleading, or deceptive claims about the efficacy, safety, or comparative benefits of non-surgical hair restoration treatments. For example, practitioners should refrain from guaranteeing "100% hair regrowth" or stating that a treatment is "completely risk-free" without evidence to support these claims. Similarly, describing a therapy as "FDA approved for hair restoration" when it is not specifically approved for this indication constitutes a misleading statement. Practitioners should also be transparent about the limitations, risks, and realistic expectations associated with each treatment option, ensuring patients can make informed decisions based on accurate and verifiable information. Hair restoration practitioners must implement appropriate safeguards to ensure the confidentiality of patient information, including secure storage and transmission of medical records, limited access to patient data, and regular staff training to remain Health Insurance Portability and Accountability Act (HIPAA) compliant.

Ethical Considerations in Hair Restoration

In addition to legal and regulatory compliance, hair restoration practitioners must also navigate a range of ethical considerations that impact patient care, professional integrity, and the reputation of the field (Atiyeh et al. 2020). The principle of non-maleficence, or avoiding harm to patients, is a cornerstone of medical ethics. Hair restoration practitioners must prioritize patient safety and well-being in all aspects of their practice, from selecting appropriate treatments and products to monitoring for adverse events and complications. This may involve carefully weighing the potential risks and benefits of each intervention, considering individual patient factors and preferences, and being prepared to adjust or discontinue treatment if necessary to prevent harm. The principle of beneficence requires practitioners to act in the best interests of their patients and to promote their welfare. This may involve recommending treatments that are most likely to be effective, safe, and well tolerated for each individual patient, based on the available scientific evidence and clinical expertise. Practitioners should also strive to provide compassionate, supportive care that addresses the emotional and psychological impacts of hair loss, as well as the physical symptoms. Providers must ensure that all patients have equitable access to care and are treated with respect, dignity, and fairness, regardless of their age, gender, race, ethnicity, sexual orientation, or socioeconomic status. This may involve addressing disparities in access to hair restoration services, providing culturally competent care, and advocating for policies that promote diversity, inclusion, and social justice in the healthcare system. Maintaining professional integrity and appropriate boundaries is essential for building trust and respect with patients and colleagues. Hair restoration practitioners must be honest, transparent, and accountable in their clinical practice, research, and business dealings. They should avoid conflicts of interest, such as accepting gifts or incentives from industry representatives that could bias their treatment recommendations or compromise their objectivity. Practitioners must also maintain appropriate professional boundaries with patients, avoiding personal or intimate relationships that could exploit the power differential or undermine the therapeutic alliance. Regular self-reflection, peer review, and ongoing education in medical ethics can help practitioners navigate the complex legal and ethical landscape of non-surgical hair restoration with skill, sensitivity, and sound judgment.

Patient Confidentiality and Consent

Protecting patient confidentiality and obtaining informed consent are two of the most critical legal and ethical obligations in non-surgical hair restoration. Practitioners must implement rigorous policies and procedures to safeguard patient privacy, ensure the security of medical records, and facilitate open, transparent communication about treatment options and expectations.

As discussed earlier, hair restoration practices must comply with HIPAA regulations for protecting the privacy and security of patient health information. This includes implementing technical, physical, and administrative safeguards to prevent unauthorized access, use, or disclosure of patient data. Practitioners should also provide regular training to staff on HIPAA requirements, as well as develop and enforce policies for reporting and responding to privacy breaches or violations. Patient privacy considerations also extend to the use of patient images, testimonials, or other personal information in marketing and advertising materials. Practitioners must obtain specific, written consent from patients before using their likeness, name, or treatment details in any public-facing content, such as websites, social media posts, or print advertisements (Marion et al. 2023). Patients should be fully informed about the nature and purpose of the marketing use, as well as their right to revoke consent at any time.
Obtaining informed consent is not a one-time event, but an ongoing process of communication and shared decision-making between the practitioner and patient. Practitioners should develop standardized informed consent forms that clearly explain the nature, purpose, benefits, risks, and alternatives to each proposed treatment, as well as the expected outcomes and long-term maintenance requirements. However, the informed consent process should also involve verbal discussion, answering patient questions, and assessing patient understanding and voluntariness.

Informed Consent Process

1. *Condition and prognosis*: Explain the patient's specific hair loss condition, whether it's androgenetic alopecia or another type of hair thinning, and what the expected course of the condition is without treatment.
2. *Proposed treatment*: Clearly describe the non-surgical treatment options (e.g., platelet-rich plasma [PRP], laser therapy, microneedling) and how they work. This should include the frequency and duration of treatment sessions, what the procedure entails, and the expected level of improvement. Discuss alternative non-surgical methods or other hair restoration options, such as topical medications (e.g., minoxidil), oral medications (e.g., finasteride), or even surgical options like hair transplantation, in case non-surgical methods are not effective.
3. *Risks*: Outline the potential risks associated with each non-surgical treatment. For example, with PRP therapy, this could include swelling, bruising, and infection. For laser therapy, potential scalp irritation may occur. These risks should be outlined in detail, while emphasizing that non-surgical hair restoration treatments generally carry minimal risks compared to more invasive procedures.
4. *Expected outcomes*: Set realistic expectations for the likely outcome of the non-surgical treatment. Patients need to understand that results may vary, and complete hair regrowth may not be achievable. The success or failure of the treatment should be discussed. Also, provide a clear timeline of the procedure, starting with the preparation, treatment sessions, and the expected time frame for seeing results.
5. *Post-treatment expectations*: Discuss what the patient can expect post-treatment, including any potential side effects like redness or discomfort, and instructions for aftercare, such as avoiding sun exposure or specific hair care practices.

6. *Costs*: Offer a detailed breakdown of the cost of the procedure, including the number of sessions needed and any follow-up treatments, as well as whether additional supportive treatments like nutritional supplements or topical solutions are recommended.

Accurate, complete, and timely documentation of the informed consent process is essential for legal and ethical compliance. Practitioners should maintain signed informed consent forms in each patient's medical record, along with detailed notes on the specific information provided, questions asked, and concerns raised during the consent discussion. Regular audits of informed consent documentation can help ensure consistency and identify areas for improvement. Obtaining informed consent for non-surgical hair restoration in minors or patients with cognitive impairments or mental illness requires additional legal and ethical safeguards. In general, practitioners should adhere to medical standards, ensure informed consent, and manage patient expectations.

Case Examples

McGlinn v. Chaffoo: This California case involved allegations of negligence during a follicular unit excision (FUE) procedure. The plaintiff claimed that unsupervised technicians improperly performed parts of the procedure, leading to injuries. The lawsuit was voluntarily dismissed in 2019, meaning there was no substantive ruling on the case's merits. However, it underscores the legal risks associated with delegating critical tasks to unqualified personnel without proper supervision. Practitioners must ensure that all staff involved in hair restoration procedures are adequately trained and supervised to avoid potential legal complications.

Salmanzadeh v. Bosley Medical Group: Bosley, a well-known hair restoration company, has faced multiple lawsuits over the years, including claims of fraud, medical malpractice, false advertising, and data breaches. In this case, a 70-year-old patient alleged that Bosley Medical Group misrepresented the nature and scope of his hair transplant procedure. The patient suffered complications and scarring, which he attributed to negligence and fraudulent claims. While the jury ruled in favor of Bosley on the negligence claim, they awarded the plaintiff $2.7 million for misrepresentation. This significant award underscores the financial and reputational risks associated with unclear or exaggerated claims. Transparency is essential in patient consultations. Practitioners must provide accurate, evidence-based information about expected outcomes, risks, and procedural details to avoid allegations of misrepresentation.

Bosley Hair Restoration cases: In a 1996 lawsuit, a patient alleged negligent surgery and misrepresentation, resulting in complications. Although the jury was divided, the Court of Appeals ultimately upheld the verdict in favor of Bosley on the fraud claim while reversing the decision on medical malpractice. The malpractice claim was sent for retrial, though the final outcome remains unknown. Maintaining high standards of medical practice and accurate marketing is critical to avoiding litigation. Misleading advertisements or overselling the efficacy of treatments can lead to legal disputes and loss of patient trust.

Conclusion

Navigating the legal and ethical complexities of non-surgical hair restoration requires a strong commitment to compliance, patient welfare, and integrity. Adhering to regulations such as FDA guidelines, licensing requirements, advertising standards, and HIPAA privacy rules ensures a safe and trustworthy practice environment. Equally important are ethical principles like non-maleficence, beneficence, justice, and transparency, which guide patient care and professional conduct. Safeguarding patient confidentiality, obtaining informed consent, and fostering open communication are fundamental to building trust and empowering patients in their treatment decisions. As the field evolves, new technologies and treatments will bring both opportunities and challenges. Practitioners must stay informed, adapt to emerging standards, and prioritize patient-centered care to remain at the forefront of this dynamic specialty. By doing so, they can ensure ethical practice while delivering innovative, effective solutions for hair restoration. The final chapter will explore the latest emerging trends shaping the future of non-surgical hair restoration.

Chapter 18

Emerging Trends and Future Directions

Julyssa A. Renteria, Robert Dorfman and Robert Greer

Introduction

As the field of non-surgical hair restoration continues to evolve and advance, it is essential for practitioners to stay informed about the latest developments, technologies, and best practices in order to provide the highest quality care to their patients. This chapter explores some of the emerging trends and future directions in non-surgical hair restoration, including new technologies and treatments, advances in regenerative medicine and cell-based therapies, the growing role of genetics and precision medicine, and the importance of ongoing research and clinical trials. By staying abreast of these developments and positioning themselves at the forefront of innovation, hair restoration practitioners can continue to expand the frontiers of what is possible in this exciting and dynamic field.

Emerging Trends and Technologies

Non-surgical hair restoration is a rapidly evolving field, with new technologies and treatments continuously emerging to improve the efficacy, safety, and accessibility of care. Some of the most promising trends and technologies on the horizon are discussed next.

Nanotechnology

Nanotechnology is rapidly advancing in the field of hair restoration, offering targeted and efficient drug delivery systems. Nanoparticles are engineered to encapsulate and deliver hair growth-promoting agents, such as finasteride or minoxidil, directly to hair follicles, reducing systemic absorption and minimizing side effects. These approaches also target specific cellular pathways involved in hair follicle cycling and regeneration, enabling more personalized treatments. Nanomaterials, including polymer-based and lipid-based nanoparticles, nanosheets, nanotubes, and inorganic nanoparticles, provide several advantages. They improve the stability and bioavailability of active compounds, ensuring consistent therapeutic effects (Pereira-Silva et al. 2022). By enabling

DOI: 10.1201/9781032726397-18

targeted delivery, nanocarriers enhance drug retention at the hair follicle site while reducing systemic side effects (Wu et al. 2024). Controlled and sustained drug release further maintains therapeutic levels over time, minimizing application frequency (Tampucci et al. 2022). Additionally, nanotechnology enhances drug penetration through the skin barrier, as seen with ultradeformable liposomes delivering hydrophilic and lipophilic agents like caffeine (Thepphankulngarm et al. 2024). Combining nanotechnology with other treatments, such as microneedling, has demonstrated synergistic effects, improving efficacy and achieving superior hair regeneration compared to conventional therapies (S. Zhang et al. 2024).

Robotic and Automated Hair Restoration Systems

While surgical hair restoration techniques, such as follicular unit extraction (FUE) and follicular unit transplantation (FUT), have traditionally been performed manually by skilled surgeons, new robotic and automated systems are emerging that may help to improve the precision, consistency, and speed of these procedures. For example, some systems use high-resolution imaging and machine learning algorithms to identify and extract individual hair follicles, while others use robotically controlled tools to create recipient sites and implant grafts with micron-level accuracy (Rose and Nusbaum 2014; Kanayama et al. 2021; Yuan et al. 2022; Bassino et al. 2015; H. Zhang et al. 2024; Pinto and Terskikh 2021; Anudeep et al. 2022; Chen et al. 2021; Wang et al. 2023). While these systems are still in the early stages of development and adoption, they may offer new possibilities for combining surgical and non-surgical approaches to hair restoration in the future (Figure 18.1).

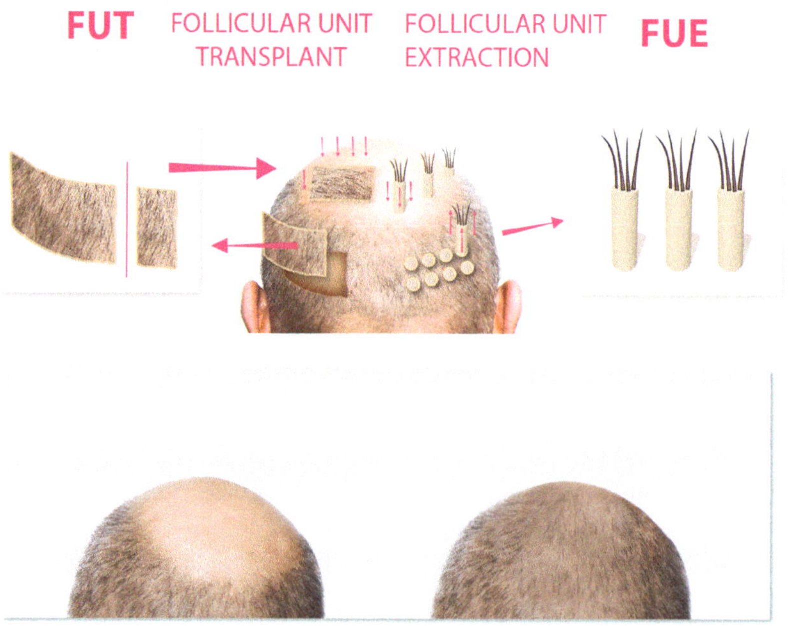

Figure 18.1 The role of robotic and automated systems in hair restoration, highlighting advancements in precision, consistency, and efficiency in procedures like follicular unit transplantation (FUT) and follicular unit extraction (FUE) (from AventusClinic.com, with permission).

Microvascular Tissue Engineering

Microvascular tissue plays a pivotal role in hair restoration by promoting perifollicular angiogenesis, which is essential for hair follicle health and growth. Enhanced vascularization around hair follicles supports their regeneration and vitality. For instance, Yuan et al. (2022) demonstrated that a microneedle patch loaded with conditioned media from hypoxia-pretreated mesenchymal stem cells boosted perifollicular vascularization and activated hair follicle stem cells, accelerating hair regeneration in an androgenetic alopecia (AGA) mouse model. Similarly, Bassino et al. (2015) highlighted the paracrine crosstalk between dermal papilla cells and microvascular endothelial cells, which fosters angiogenesis and supports hair follicle development. This approach highlights the direct role of microvascular tissue in creating an optimal environment for hair follicle survival and regeneration.

An emerging innovation in this field involves the use of mVASC, a product leveraging microvascular tissue for therapeutic purposes. mVASC is a ready-to-use product derived from human cadaveric subcutaneous tissue, processed and lyophilized into a 19.5 mm diameter disk embedded with a cryopreservative and crystalloid. The structural properties of this microvascular extracellular matrix (ECM) are designed to enhance tissue repair by promoting angiogenesis and restoring blood flow. mVASC is FDA approved for treating deficiencies in microvasculature and has shown potential in conditions involving compromised circulation, including diabetic foot ulcers.

Preclinical Data Supporting mVASC

mVASC demonstrated superior vascular reconstruction in a mouse model of ischemia-reperfusion injury. Mice treated with mVASC displayed nearly complete restoration of blood flow in ischemic limbs by day 14 compared to control animals. The mean perfusion ratio in mVASC-treated animals reached 82% of the contralateral control limb, significantly higher than the 59% observed in control animals. This robust revascularization prevented tissue necrosis and highlights the potential for mVASC to restore microvascular integrity in ischemic tissues. In a mouse model of pressure ulcers, mVASC significantly accelerated wound closure and improved healing metrics. Topical application of mVASC resulted in an increased mean closure rate from day 5 through day 13, with 92% closure observed in mVASC-treated ulcers versus 38% in controls by day 13. The treatment also expedited scab removal and raised skin temperature, consistent with enhanced blood flow and improved microvascular function. mVASC significantly enhanced blood vessel formation in a SCID mouse model. Treated Matrigel plugs demonstrated a 33% to 139% increase in vessel ingrowth compared to controls, with a notable rise in medium-sized and large-diameter vessels. These results suggest that mVASC promotes both the quantity and maturity of new blood vessels, which are essential for sustained tissue regeneration.

Clinical Data Supporting mVASC

The HIFLO (High-Flow Oxygenation) trial demonstrated the efficacy of mVASC in treating diabetic foot ulcers, highlighting its potential for promoting vascular and tissue repair. This randomized controlled trial compared weekly applications of mVASC with standard wound care, showing significantly higher rates of complete wound closure and improved blood flow in the mVASC group. Laser Doppler imaging confirmed robust vascular regeneration, with perfusion levels near those of healthy tissues by the study's conclusion. Patients also experienced reduced pain, improved sensation, and enhanced nerve function, supported by histological findings of increased angiogenesis, nerve regeneration, and reduced inflammation. mVASC was well-tolerated, with no serious adverse events reported. These results underscore mVASC's ability to restore microvascular function and durable tissue repair, suggesting potential applications in hair restoration, where perifollicular vascularization is essential for follicle health and growth. Although further studies are needed, the mechanisms demonstrated in this trial provide a promising foundation for treating vascular-related hair loss conditions.

Advances in three-dimensional (3D) culture systems and biomaterials have enhanced the potential for hair follicle regeneration by providing an in vivo-like environment for dermal papilla cells (DPCs) and hair follicle stem cells (HFSCs). Zheng and Xu (2023) emphasized the role of ECM-mimicking scaffolds in maintaining cell homeostasis and promoting epithelial–mesenchymal interactions, critical for hair follicle regeneration. Similarly, Liu et al. (2023) developed an optimized 3D co-culture system that restored the hair-inductive properties of human dermal papilla cells, showing improved outcomes compared to traditional 2D cultures.

Stemson Therapeutics is at the forefront of hair restoration research, leveraging induced pluripotent stem cells (iPSCs) to address the limitations of current hair restoration methods. By reprogramming somatic cells into iPSCs, Stemson has developed a method to differentiate these cells into the various types required for hair follicle formation, such as dermal papilla and epithelial cells. This innovative approach offers the potential to create new hair follicles de novo, providing an unlimited source of folliculogenic cells for transplantation. This technology could transform the treatment landscape for patients with advanced hair loss, particularly those without sufficient donor hair for transplantation.

Research published by Wang et al. (2023) revealed a significant connection between senescent melanocytes in melanocytic nevi and enhanced hair growth. The study demonstrated that these senescent cells secrete osteopontin, a signaling molecule that activates epithelial HFSCs, driving them out of dormancy and into the growth phase. This process results in robust hair renewal, providing new insights into hair follicle biology and regeneration. Using murine models for congenital and acquired nevi, the researchers found that the accumulation of senescent melanocytes in the dermis triggered the activation of HFSCs and induced ectopic anagen (growth) phases in nearby hair follicles. Further experiments highlighted the critical role of osteopontin, as mice lacking either osteopontin (Spp1 knockout) or its receptor CD44 showed significantly reduced hair growth in response to senescent melanocytes. Injection of osteopontin into the dermis was sufficient to replicate these effects, underscoring its central role in mediating hair follicle activation. In human studies, elevated osteopontin levels were observed in pigmented nevi associated with excessive hair growth, suggesting that this mechanism is conserved across species. The findings redefine the role of senescent cells, which are traditionally linked to aging and tissue degeneration, showing their capacity to enhance regeneration in specific contexts. This discovery opens the door to novel therapeutic approaches in hair restoration, such as targeting senescent cell secretomes or modulating osteopontin-CD44 signaling to promote hair growth.

Hair Cloning

Hair cloning, also referred to as follicular cell implantation or hair follicle neogenesis, represents an innovative and potentially transformative approach to hair restoration, particularly for addressing AGA (Higgins and Christiano 2014; Anudeep et al. 2022). Unlike current treatments, such as topical estrogens, ketoconazole, finasteride, minoxidil, and polytherapy, which primarily work by modulating androgen levels, promoting blood flow, or reducing inflammation, hair cloning seeks to overcome their major limitation, the inability to generate new hair follicles. The concept of hair cloning dates back to the 1960s when researchers first began exploring methods to replicate hair follicles for transplantation. Early efforts were hampered by limited understanding of follicular biology and the technological constraints of the time. By the 1990s, advancements in tissue engineering reignited interest in hair cloning, with researchers focusing on isolating and cultivating dermal papilla cells, the specialized structures critical for hair follicle formation. Over the decades, two primary approaches to hair cloning have emerged: in vivo (within the body) cloning and in vitro (in the lab) cloning. While both hold promise, each comes with unique methodologies, advantages, and challenges.

1. *In vivo hair cloning*: This approach involves replicating hair follicles directly within the body. It typically entails harvesting healthy hair follicle cells and implanting them into the scalp, where they stimulate nearby follicles to regenerate or induce the formation of new ones. This method leverages the natural environment of the scalp to support follicular growth. One major advantage of in vivo cloning is that it bypasses some of the complexities associated with cultivating cells in a lab environment. However, challenges include ensuring consistent integration of implanted cells and achieving cosmetically acceptable outcomes.
2. *In vitro hair cloning*: In vitro cloning involves culturing hair follicle cells, such as dermal papilla and keratinocyte cells, in a laboratory setting. These cells are expanded and multiplied in a petri dish before being implanted into balding areas of the scalp to induce new follicle growth. This method offers greater control over cell preparation and quality but faces significant hurdles, including ensuring the survival of implanted cells, avoiding immune rejection, and standardizing outcomes across patients. In vitro cloning also requires sophisticated cell culture techniques and precise microenvironmental conditions to maintain the inductive properties of the cells (Figure 18.2).

Advances in Regenerative Medicine

Regenerative medicine is a rapidly evolving field that seeks to harness the body's own healing and regenerative capabilities to treat a wide range of diseases and conditions, including hair loss. Some of the most promising advances in regenerative medicine for hair restoration are explained in this section.

The extracellular matrix is a complex network of proteins, glycoproteins, and other molecules that provide structural and biochemical support to cells and tissues. In regenerative medicine, ECM-derived materials and other scaffolding technologies are being explored as a way to create a supportive microenvironment for cell growth and tissue regeneration. In the context of hair restoration, some researchers are investigating the use of ECM-based scaffolds or hydrogels (X. Zhang et al. 2019; Chen et al. 2020; Kang et al. 2023) to deliver growth factors, stem cells, or other therapeutic agents to the scalp, potentially enhancing their effects on hair follicle regeneration and cycling.

Gene therapy involves the introduction of new genes or the modification of existing genes to treat or prevent disease. In the context of hair restoration, gene therapy approaches may involve delivering genes that encode hair growth-promoting factors, such as Wnt proteins or prostaglandin D2 receptor antagonists, to the scalp using viral or non-viral vectors (Ma et al. 2022). Another related approach is epigenetic modulation, which involves altering the expression of genes without changing the underlying DNA sequence. For example, some studies have suggested that modulating the activity of histone deacetylases (HDACs) or DNA methyltransferases (DNMTs) could help to promote hair follicle stem cell activation and regeneration.

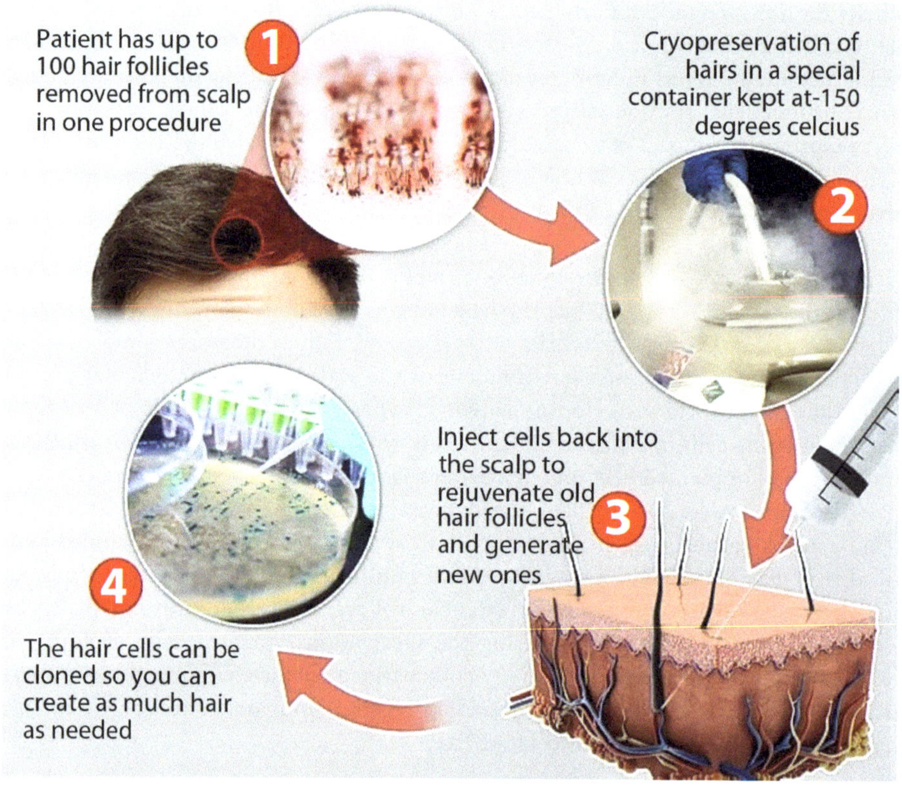

Figure 18.2 The process of hair cloning, a cutting-edge approach to hair restoration aimed at overcoming the limitations of conventional treatments for androgenetic alopecia (AGA) (from HairDr.com, with permission).

The Role of Genetics and Precision Medicine

Genetics and precision medicine are playing an increasingly important role in the diagnosis, treatment, and prevention of hair loss. By understanding the genetic and molecular basis of different types of alopecia, practitioners can develop more targeted and personalized approaches to hair restoration that take into account each patient's unique biology and risk factors.

Some of the key ways in which genetics and precision medicine are shaping the future of hair restoration include:

1. *Genetic testing and risk assessment*: Genetic testing is becoming more widely available and affordable, allowing practitioners to assess a patient's risk of developing certain types of hair loss based on their genetic profile. For example, variations in genes such as the androgen receptor (AR) gene and the aromatase (CYP19A1) gene have been associated with an increased risk of androgenetic alopecia in both men and women (Keene and Goren 2011). By identifying patients with high-risk genotypes, practitioners can offer earlier and more targeted interventions to prevent or slow the progression of hair loss.
2. *Pharmacogenomics and personalized treatment*: Pharmacogenomics is the study of how genetic variations influence an individual's response to drugs. In the context of hair restoration,

pharmacogenomic testing could help practitioners to predict which patients are most likely to benefit from or experience side effects from certain medications, such as finasteride or minoxidil. This information could be used to tailor treatment regimens to each patient's unique genetic profile, potentially improving efficacy and reducing the risk of adverse events.

3. *Targeted therapies for specific molecular pathways*: As our understanding of the molecular mechanisms underlying hair loss continues to grow, researchers are developing new targeted therapies that can modulate specific pathways or molecules involved in hair follicle cycling and regeneration. For example, some studies have identified small molecule inhibitors of the Janus kinase (JAK) family of enzymes as potential treatments for alopecia areata, an autoimmune form of hair loss. Other targets being explored include the Wnt/β-catenin pathway, the transforming growth factor-β (TGF-β) pathway, and the prostaglandin D2 receptor (GPR44) (Dey-Rao and Sinha 2017).
4. *Precision medicine approaches to hair transplantation*: While hair transplantation is a surgical procedure, advances in precision medicine are also influencing this field. For example, some researchers are exploring the use of gene expression profiling or other molecular diagnostics to identify the optimal donor and recipient sites for hair follicle grafts, based on factors such as the expression of hair growth-related genes or the presence of certain cell types. Other approaches may involve the use of 3D printing or other advanced manufacturing techniques to create customized hair follicle scaffolds or delivery systems for growth factors and other therapeutic agents.

It is important to note that many of these approaches are still in the early stages of research and development, and more studies will be needed to fully validate their safety and efficacy in the clinical setting.

The Importance of Research and Clinical Trials

Ongoing research and clinical trials are essential for advancing the field of non-surgical hair restoration and ensuring that patients have access to the safest, most effective, and evidence-based treatments available. Some of the key reasons why research and clinical trials are so important in hair restoration include:

1. *Validating the safety and efficacy of new treatments*: Before any new hair restoration treatment can be widely adopted in clinical practice, it must undergo rigorous testing in preclinical and clinical studies to demonstrate its safety and efficacy. Clinical trials, in particular, are essential for evaluating the performance of new treatments in real-world patient populations, identifying potential side effects or limitations, and comparing their effectiveness to existing standards of care. By participating in or following the results of these trials, practitioners can gain a more complete and objective understanding of the risks and benefits of different treatment options.
2. *Improving our understanding of hair biology and pathology*: Research studies that investigate the basic biology of hair follicles, the mechanisms of hair loss, and the factors that influence hair growth and cycling are essential for developing new and more effective treatments for hair restoration. For example, studies that elucidate the role of stem cells, growth factors, and other signaling molecules in hair follicle regeneration may lead to the development of new regenerative therapies or drug targets. Similarly, studies that explore the genetic and

epigenetic factors that contribute to different types of alopecia may help to identify new biomarkers or risk factors that could be used for early diagnosis or personalized treatment.

3. *Driving innovation and technological development*: Clinical trials and research studies are also important drivers of innovation and technological development in the field of hair restoration. As new treatments and technologies emerge, they must be rigorously tested and validated in order to gain regulatory approval and widespread adoption. By participating in these studies or providing feedback on their experiences with new treatments, practitioners can help to shape the direction of innovation and ensure that new technologies are safe, effective, and practical for use in the clinical setting.
4. *Advancing evidence-based practice and patient care*: Ultimately, the goal of research and clinical trials in hair restoration is to advance evidence-based practice and improve patient care. By staying informed about the latest research developments and incorporating them into their clinical decision-making, practitioners can provide their patients with the most up-to-date and scientifically sound treatment options.

To stay informed about the latest research and clinical trials in hair restoration, practitioners can attend scientific conferences, read peer-reviewed journals, participate in professional societies and research networks, and collaborate with academic or industry partners. Practitioners may consider participating in clinical trials themselves, either as investigators or by referring patients to ongoing studies. By actively engaging with the research community and contributing to the growing body of knowledge in hair restoration, you can help to shape the future of the field and provide the best possible care to your patients.

Conclusion

As we come to the end of this final chapter, we understand that the field of non-surgical hair restoration is rapidly advancing, with innovations such as advanced laser therapies, nanoparticle drug delivery, regenerative medicine, and precision tools offering new possibilities. Practitioners must stay informed, critically evaluate emerging treatments, and integrate evidence-based innovations into clinical practice to optimize patient care. Ongoing research and clinical trials are essential for validating new approaches and advancing the field. By engaging with the research community, staying updated on studies, and contributing insights, practitioners can help shape the future of hair restoration, ensuring patients have access to safe and effective treatments.

Ultimately, the goal of hair restoration practice is to provide the best possible care to our patients, to help them achieve their desired outcomes, and to improve their overall quality of life. By staying at the forefront of this exciting and dynamic field, by continuously learning and adapting to new developments, and by always putting the needs and well-being of our patients first, we can achieve this goal and make a meaningful difference in the lives of those affected by hair loss.

As we look to the future of non-surgical hair restoration, let us embrace the challenges and opportunities that lie ahead, and work together as a community of practitioners, researchers, and innovators to advance the field and provide the highest quality care to our patients.

Afterword

As we come to the end of this comprehensive guide to non-surgical hair restoration, I am filled with a sense of excitement and optimism for the future of our field. Over the course of this book, we have explored the fundamental principles of hair biology and pathology; the various non-surgical treatment modalities and their underlying mechanisms of action; and the practical strategies for patient evaluation, treatment planning, and long-term management.

We have also delved into the complex legal and ethical considerations surrounding hair restoration practice, and the importance of effective communication, patient education, and expectation management in building a successful and rewarding career in this field.

Throughout this journey, I have shared my clinical experiences, insights, and lessons learned in the hope of providing a valuable resource and reference for practitioners at all stages of their careers. As a passionate advocate for evidence-based, patient-centered care in hair restoration, my goal has been to empower readers with the knowledge, skills, and tools they need to provide the highest quality care to their patients and to navigate the challenges and opportunities of this dynamic field with confidence and integrity.

Looking ahead, I am excited to see how the field of non-surgical hair restoration will continue to evolve and advance in the coming years. With the rapid pace of scientific discovery and technological innovation, I have no doubt that we will see many new and groundbreaking treatments and approaches emerge, from regenerative therapies and precision medicine tools to advanced imaging and diagnostic technologies.

At the same time, I believe that the fundamental principles and values that have guided our field thus far will continue to serve as the bedrock of our practice: a deep commitment to patient safety and well-being, a rigorous approach to evidence-based medicine, a collaborative and multidisciplinary spirit, and a passion for lifelong learning and professional growth.

As we navigate the challenges and opportunities of the future, I encourage all of my colleagues in hair restoration to stay curious, to stay engaged, and to stay committed to the highest standards of care and integrity. Together, we can continue to push the boundaries of what is possible in this field and to make a meaningful difference in the lives of the patients we serve.

Thank you for joining me on this journey through the world of non-surgical hair restoration. I hope that this book has been a valuable and informative resource for you, and that it has inspired you to continue learning, growing, and making a positive impact in this exciting and rewarding field.

With gratitude and best wishes,
Dr. Robert Dorfman, Done by Dorfman, Beverly Hills

References

Abaci HE, Coffman A, Doucet Y, Chen J, Jackōw J, Wang E, Guo Z, Shin JU, Jahoda CA, Christiano AM. Tissue engineering of human hair follicles using a biomimetic developmental approach. *Nat Commun.* 2018;9(1):5301.

Abdel-Rahman SM, Nahata MC, Powell DA. Response to initial griseofulvin therapy in pediatric patients with tinea capitis. *Ann Pharmacother.* 1997;31(4):406–10.

Ablon G. A 6-month, randomized, double-blind, placebo-controlled study evaluating the ability of a marine complex supplement to promote hair growth in men with thinning hair. J Cosmet Dermatol. 2016;15(4):358–66.

Acosta L, Byham-Gray L, Kurzer M, Samavat H. Hepatotoxicity with high-dose green tea extract: Effect of catechol-O-methyltransferase and uridine 5'-diphospho-glucuronosyltransferase 1A4 genotypes. *J Diet Suppl.* 2023;20(6):850–69.

Afiune LAF, Ushirobira CY, Barbosa DPP, de Souza PEN, Leles MIG, Cunha-Filho M, et al. Novel iron oxide nanocarriers loading finasteride or dutasteride: Enhanced skin penetration for topical treatment of alopecia. *Int J Pharm.* 2020;587:119709.

Alhattab MK, Al Abdullah MJ, Al-Janabi MH, Aljanaby WA, Alwakeel HA. The effect of 1540-nm fractional erbium-glass laser in the treatment of androgenic alopecia. *J Cosmet Dermatol.* 2020;19(4):878–83.

Akbarnejad F. The role of green tea (Camellia sinensis) in the management of Androgenetic Alopecia (AGA): A review. *Int J Multidisciplinary Res Growth Eval.* 2023;4(05):308–16.

Ali AK, Heran BS, Etminan M. Persistent sexual dysfunction and suicidal ideation in young men treated with low-dose finasteride: A pharmacovigilance study. *Pharmacotherapy.* 2015;35(7):687–95.

Ali ST, Feldman SR. Patient satisfaction in dermatology: A qualitative assessment. *Dermatol Online J.* 2014;20(2). https://doi.org/10.5070/D3202021534.

Allen HB, Honig PJ, Leyden JJ, McGinley KJ. Selenium sulfide: Adjunctive therapy for tinea capitis. *Pediatrics.* 1982;69(1):81–3

Almohanna HM, Ahmed AA, Tsatalis JP, Tosti A. The role of vitamins and minerals in hair loss: A review. *Dermatol Ther (Heidelb).* 2019;9(1):51–70.

Alonso LC, Rosenfield RL. Molecular genetic and endocrine mechanisms of hair growth. *Horm Res.* 2003;60:1–13.

Alser OH, Goutos I. The evidence behind the use of platelet-rich plasma (PRP) in scar management: A literature review. *Scars Burn Heal.* 2018;4:2059513118808773.

Altomare G, Capella GL. Depression circumstantially related to the administration of finasteride for androgenetic alopecia. *J Dermatol.* 2002;29(10):665–9.

Alves R, Grimalt R. Platelet-rich plasma in combination with 5% minoxidil topical solution and 1 mg oral finasteride for the treatment of androgenetic alopecia: A randomized placebo-controlled, double-blind, half-head study. *Dermatol Surg.* 2018;44(1):126–30.

Amara S, Abdelmelek H, Garrel C, Guiraud P, Douki T, Ravanat JL, Favier A, Sakly M, Ben Rhouma K. Preventive effect of zinc against cadmium-induced oxidative stress in the rat testis. *J Reprod Dev.* 2008;54(2):129–34.

American Psychiatric Association. *Diagnostic and statistical manual of mental disorders: DSM-5.* 5th edn. Arlington, VA: American Psychiatric Publishing; 2013.

Anastassakis K. Saw palmetto (Serenoa repens Sabal serrulatum). In: *Androgenetic alopecia from A to Z*. Cham: Springer; 2022. https://doi.org/10.1007/978-3-031-08057-9_49.

Anderi R, Makdissy N, Azar A, Rizk F, Hamade A. Cellular therapy with human autologous adipose-derived adult cells of stromal vascular fraction for alopecia areata. *Stem Cell Res Ther.* 2018;9(1):141.

Anderson RJ, Kudlacek PE, Clemens DL. Sulfation of minoxidil by multiple human cytosolic sulfotransferases. *Chem Biol Interact.* 1998;109(1–3):53–67.

Andrade JFM, Matos BN, Rocho RV, Barbalho GN, Cunha-Filho M, Gelfuso GM, et al. Evaluation of dutasteride-loaded liposomes and transfersomes for follicular-targeting for androgenic alopecia topical treatment. *Pharmaceutics.* 2024;16(12):1524.

Ankad BS, Beergouder SL, Moodalgiri VM. Lichen planopilaris versus discoid lupus erythematosus: A trichoscopic perspective. *Int J Trichology.* 2013;5(4):204–7.

Anudeep TC, Jeyaraman M, Muthu S, Rajendran RL, Gangadaran P, Mishra PC, Sharma S, Jha SK, Ahn BC. Advancing regenerative cellular therapies in non-scarring alopecia. *Pharmaceutics.* 2022;14(3):612.

Arck PC, Handjiski B, Peters EMJ, Peter AS, Hagen E, Fischer A, Klapp BF, Paus R. Stress inhibits hair growth in mice by induction of premature catagen development and deleterious perifollicular inflammatory events via neuropeptide substance P-dependent pathways. *Am J Pathol.* 2003;162(3):803–14.

Asghar F, Shamim N, Farooque U, Sheikh H, Aqeel R. Telogen effluvium: A review of the literature. *Cureus.* 2020;12(5):e8320.

Asilian A, Farmani A, Saber M. Clinical efficacy and safety of low-dose oral minoxidil versus topical solution in the improvement of androgenetic alopecia: A randomized controlled trial. *J Cosmet Dermatol.* 2024;23(3):949–57.

Atiyeh BS, Rubeiz MT, Hayek SN. Aesthetic/cosmetic surgery and ethical challenges. *Aesthetic Plast Surg.* 2020;44(4):1364–74.

Aukerman EL, Jafferany M. The psychological consequences of androgenetic alopecia: A systematic review. *J Cosmet Dermatol.* 2023;22(1):89–95.

Avci P, Gupta GK, Clark J, Wikonkal N, Hamblin MR. Low-level laser (light) therapy (LLLT) for treatment of hair loss. *Lasers Surg Med.* 2014;Feb;46(2):144–51. doi: 10.1002/lsm.22170.

Avram MR, Cole JP, Gandelman M, Haber R, Knudsen R, Leavitt MT, Leonard RT Jr, Puig CJ, Rose PT, Vogel JE, Ziering CL. The potential role of minoxidil in the hair transplantation setting. *Dermatol Surg.* 2002;28(10):894–900.

Babadjouni A, Reddy M, Zhang R, Raffi J, Phong C, Mesinkovska N. Melatonin and the human hair follicle. *J Drugs Dermatol.* 2023;22(3):260–4.

Badran KW, Sand JP. Platelet-rich plasma for hair loss: Review of methods and results. *Facial Plast Surg Clin North Am.* 2018;26(4):469–85.

Bailey AM, Antonovich D. Suture localization of scalp biopsy sites. *JAAD Online* 2022;87:1e1–e2.

Bains P, Kaur S, Kaur K. Comparison of dermoscopic findings in female androgenetic alopecia and telogen effluvium and female controls in a tertiary care center. *J Clin Aesthet Dermatol.* 2022;15(5):29–34.

Bak DH, Lee E, Choi MJ, Lee BC, Kwon TR, Kim JH, Jeon ES, Oh W, Mun SK, Park BC, Na J, Kim BJ. Protective effects of human umbilical cord blood-derived mesenchymal stem cells against dexamethasone-induced apoptotic cell death in hair follicles. *Int J Mol Med.* 2020;45(2):556–68.

Bank J, Feingold RS, Korn P, Light D, Israeli R. Branding a plastic surgery group practice: A case study. *Plast Reconstr Surg.* 2023;152(1):188e–95e.

Bassino E, Gasparri F, Giannini V, Munaron L. Paracrine crosstalk between human hair follicle dermal papilla cells and microvascular endothelial cells. *Exp Dermatol.* 2015;24(5):388–90.

Bauman Medical. PRP Platelet-Rich Plasma + ACell + ECMs. Accessed July 1, 2025. Available from: https://www.baumanmedical.com/hair-restoration-options/prp-platelet-rich-plasma-acell-ecms/

Benincá JP, et al. Analysis of the anti-inflammatory properties of Rosmarinus officinalis L. in mice. Food Chem. 2011;124(2):468–75.

Bennett ML, Fleischer AB, Loveless JW, Feldman SR. Oral griseofulvin remains the treatment of choice for tinea capitis in children. *Pediatr Dermatol.* 2000;17(4):304–9.

Berger RS, Fu JL, Smiles KA, et al. The effects of minoxidil, 1% pyrithione zinc and a combination of both on hair density: A randomized controlled trial. *Br J Dermatol.* 2003;149(2):354–62.

Bertin ACJ, Vilarinho A, Junqueira ALA. Fractional non-ablative laser-assisted drug delivery leads to improvement in male and female pattern hair loss. *J Cosmet Laser Ther.* 2018;20(7–8):391–4.
Billero V, Miteva M. Traction alopecia: The root of the problem. *Clin Cosmet Investig Dermatol.* 2018;11:149–59.
Bin Rubaian NF, Alzamami HFA, Amir BA. An overview of commonly used natural alternatives for the treatment of androgenetic alopecia, with special emphasis on rosemary oil. *Clin Cosmet Investig Dermatol.* 2024;17:2495–503.
Birch MP, Lalla SC, Messenger AG. Female pattern hair loss. *Clin Exp Dermatol.* 2002;27:383–8.
Birch MP, Messenger JF, Messenger AG. Hair density, hair diameter and the prevalence of female pattern hair loss. *Br J Dermatol.* 2001;144:297–304.
Birder LA, Kanai AJ, de Groat WC, Kiss S, Nealen ML, Burke NE, Dineley KE, Watkins S, Reynolds IJ, Caterina MJ. Vanilloid receptor expression suggests a sensory role for urinary bladder epithelial cells. *Proc Natl Acad Sci USA.* 2001;98(23):13396–401.
Bloch LD, Goshiyama AM, Dario MF, Escudeiro CC, Sarruf FD, Velasco MVR, Valente NYS. Chemical and physical treatments damage Caucasian and Afro-ethnic hair fibre: Analytical and image assays. *J Eur Acad Dermatol Venereol.* 2019;33(11):2158–67.
Blumer JL. Pharmacologic basis for the treatment of tinea capitis. *Pediatr Infect Dis J.* 1999;18(2):191–9.
Boersma IH, Oranje AP, Grimalt R, Iorizzo M, Piraccini BM, Verdonschot EH. The effectiveness of finasteride and dutasteride used for 3 years in women with androgenetic alopecia. *Indian J Dermatol Venereol Leprol.* 2014;80(6):521–5.
Bowman CJ, Barlow NJ, Turner KJ, Wallace DG, Foster PM. Effects of in utero exposure to finasteride on androgen-dependent reproductive development in the male rat. *Toxicol Sci.* 2003;74(2):393–406.
Brough K, Torgerson R. Hormonal therapy in female pattern hair loss. *Int J Womens Dermatol.* 2017;3:53–7.
Callender VD, Wright DR, Davis EC, Sperling LC. Hair breakage as a presenting sign of early or occult central centrifugal cicatricial alopecia: Clinicopathologic findings in 9 patients. *Arch Dermatol.* 2012;148(9):1047–52.
Carbin BE, Larsson B, Lindahl O. Treatment of benign prostatic hyperplasia with phytosterols. *Br J Urol.* 1990;66(6):639–41.
Carmina E, Azziz R, Bergfeld W, Escobar-Morreale HF, Futterweit W, Huddleston H, et al. Female pattern hair loss and androgen excess: a report from the multidisciplinary androgen excess and PCOS committee. J Clin Endocrinol Metab. 2019;104(7):2875–91.
Caserini M, Radicioni M, Leuratti C, Annoni O, Palmieri R. A novel finasteride 0.25% topical solution for androgenetic alopecia: Pharmacokinetics and effects on plasma androgen levels in healthy male volunteers. *Int J Clin Pharmacol Ther.* 2014;52(10):842–9.
Ceruti JM, Leirós GJ, Balañá ME. Androgens and androgen receptor action in skin and hair follicles. *Mol Cell Endocrinol.* 2018;465:122–33.
Chang IA, Wells MW, Chang IA, Arquette CP, Tang CJ, Gatherwright JR, Furnas HJ. The positive patient experience: A comprehensive analysis of plastic surgery online reviews. *Aesthetic Surg J.* 2022;42(9):1083–93.
Chen CH, Jiang SS, Chang IS, Wen HJ, Sun CW, Wang SL. Association between fetal exposure to phthalate endocrine disruptors and genome-wide DNA methylation at birth. *Environ Res.* 2018 Apr;162:261–70.
Chen D, Yu F, Wang C, et al. Anti-hair loss effect of a shampoo containing caffeine and adenosine. *J Cosmet Dermatol.* 2024;23:2927–33.
Chen L, Zhang J, Wang L, Wang H, Chen B. The efficacy and safety of finasteride combined with topical minoxidil for androgenetic alopecia: A systematic review and meta-analysis. *Aesthetic Plast Surg.* 2020;44(3):962–70.
Chen P, Miao Y, Zhang F, Fan Z, Huang J, Mao X, Chen J, Hu Z, Wang J. Tissue engineering ECM-enriched controllable vascularized human microtissue for hair regenerative medicine using a biomimetic developmental approach. *J Adv Res.* 2021;38:77–89.
Chen Y, Huang J, Chen R, Yang L, Wang J, Liu B, Du L, Yi Y, Jia J, Xu Y, Chen Q, Ngondi DG, Miao Y, Hu Z. Sustained release of dermal papilla-derived extracellular vesicles from injectable microgel promotes hair growth. *Theranostics.* 2020;10(3):1454–78.

Chien WY, Huang HM, Kang YN, Chen KH, Chen C. Stem cell-derived conditioned medium for alopecia: A systematic review and meta-analysis. *J Plast Reconstr Aesthet Surg.* 2024;88:182–92.

Chien Yin GO, Siong-See JL, Wang ECE. Telogen effluvium – a review of the science and current obstacles. J Dermatol Sci. 2021;101(3):156–63.

Cho SB, Goo BL, Zheng Z, Yoo KH, Kang JS, Kim H. Therapeutic efficacy and safety of a 1927-nm fractionated thulium laser on pattern hair loss: An evaluator-blinded, split-scalp study. *Lasers Med Sci.* 2018;33(4):851–9.

Cho YH, Lee SY, Jeong DW, Choi EJ, Kim YJ, Lee JG, et al. Effect of pumpkin seed oil on hair growth in men with androgenetic alopecia: a randomized, double-blind, placebo-controlled trial. Evid Based Complement Alternat Med. 2014;2014:549721.

Cho SB, Zheng Z, Kang JS, et al. Therapeutic efficacy of 1,927-nm fractionated thulium laser energy and polydeoxyribonucleotide on pattern hair loss. *Med Lasers.* 2016;5:22.

Choi N, Hwang J, Kim DY, Kim J, Song SY, Sung JH. Involvement of DKK1 secreted from adipose-derived stem cells in alopecia areata. *Cell Prolif.* 2024;57(3):e13562.

Choi YH, Cho SY, Cho IR. The different reduction rate of prostate-specific antigen in dutasteride and finasteride. *Korean J Urol.* 2010;51(10):704–8.

Chon SY, Suh DH, Liao W, et al. Chemotherapy-induced alopecia. *J Am Acad Dermatol.* 2012;67(1):e37–47.

Chu S, Foulad DP, Atanaskova Mesinkovska N. Safety profile for microneedling: A systematic review. *Dermatol Surg.* 2021;47(9):1249–54.

Chu TW, Santos L, McElwee KJ. Biology of the hair follicle and mechanisms of nonscarring and scarring alopecia. *Semin Cutan Med Surg.* 2021;40(1):43–57.

Chung H, Dai T, Sharma SK, Huang YY, Carroll JD, Hamblin MR. The nuts and bolts of low-level laser (light) therapy. Ann Biomed Eng. 2012;40(2):516–33.

Chung HJ, Goldberg LJ. Histologic features of chronic cutaneous lupus erythematosus of the scalp using horizontal sectioning: Emphasis on follicular findings. *J Am Acad Dermatol.* 2017;77(2):349–55.

Clark RV, Hermann DJ, Cunningham GR, Wilson TH, Morrill BB, Hobbs S. Marked suppression of dihydrotestosterone in men with benign prostatic hyperplasia by dutasteride, a dual 5α-reductase inhibitor. *J Clin Endocrinol Metab.* 2004;89(5):2179–84.

Clemmensen OJ, Hainau B, Hansted B. The ultrastructure of the transition zone between specialized cells ("Flügelzellen") of Huxley's layer of the inner root sheath and cells of the outer root sheath of the human hair follicle. *Am J Dermatopathol.* 1991;13(3):264–70.

Cohen B, Cadesky A, Jaggi S. Dermatologic manifestations of thyroid disease: A literature review. *Front Endocrinol.* 2023;14:1167890.

Concha JSS, Werth VP. Alopecias in lupus erythematosus. Lupus Sci Med. 2018;5(1):e000291.

Coneac A, Muresan A, Orasan MS. Antiandrogenic therapy with cyproterone acetate in female patients who suffer from both androgenetic alopecia and acne vulgaris. *Clujul Med.* 2014;87(4):226–34.

Conic RRZ, Piliang M, Bergfeld W, Atanaskova-Mesinkovska N. Vitamin D status in scarring and nonscarring alopecia. *J Am Acad Dermatol.* 2021;85(2):478–80.

Craighead DH, Alexander LM. Topical menthol increases cutaneous blood flow. *Microvasc Res.* 2016;107:39–45.

Dabek RJ, Austen WG Jr, Bojovic B. Laser-assisted hair regrowth: Fractional laser modalities for the treatment of androgenic alopecia. *Plast Reconstr Surg Glob Open.* 2019;7(4):e2157.

Dahabreh D, Jung S, Renert-Yuval Y, Bar J, Del Duca E, Guttman-Yassky E. Alopecia areata: Current treatments and new directions. *Am J Clin Dermatol.* 2023;24(6):895–912.

Dawber RP, Rundegren J. Hypertrichosis in females applying minoxidil topical solution and in normal controls. *J Eur Acad Dermatol Venereol.* 2003;17(3):271–5.

Day RM, Suzuki YJ. Cell proliferation, reactive oxygen, and cellular glutathione. *Dose Response.* 2006;3(3):425–42.

de Berker D, Dawber RP. Monilethrix treated with oral retinoids. *Clin Exp Dermatol.* 1991;16(3):226–8.

De Brouwer B, Tételin C, Leroy T, Bonfils A, Van Neste D. A controlled study of the effects of RU58841, a non-steroidal antiandrogen, on human hair production by balding scalp grafts maintained on testosterone-conditioned nude mice. *Br J Dermatol.* 1997;137(5):699–702.

Desai K, Miteva M. Recent insight on the management of lupus erythematosus alopecia. *Clin Cosmet Investig Dermatol.* 2021;14:333–47.

Desai S. A single-center study evaluating Alma TED™ and a peptide-based topical hair care formula for female and male pattern hair loss [internet], Alma Lasers, 2023. https://almalasers.com/wp-content/uploads/2023/06/Alma-TED-Desai-White-Paper-FIN_.pdf.

Dey-Rao R, Sinha AA. A genomic approach to susceptibility and pathogenesis leads to identifying potential novel therapeutic targets in androgenetic alopecia. *Genomics.* 2017;109(3–4):165–76.

Dhurat R, Chitallia J, May TW, Jayaraaman AM, Madhukara J, Anandan S, Vaidya P, Klenk A. An open-label randomized multicenter study assessing the noninferiority of a caffeine-based topical liquid 0.2% versus minoxidil 5% solution in male androgenetic alopecia. *Skin Pharmacol Physiol.* 2017;30(6):298–305.

Dhurat R, Sharma A, Rudnicka L, Kroumpouzos G, Kassir M, Galadari H, et al. 5-Alpha reductase inhibitors in androgenetic alopecia: Shifting paradigms, current concepts, comparative efficacy, and safety. *Dermatol Ther.* 2020;33(3):e13379.

Dhurat R, Shukla D, Agrawal S, Chitalia J, Ghate S, Jage M. Tinea capitis presenting as diffuse hair loss and significance of trichoscopy: Four case reports. *Skin Appendage Disord.* 2021;7(4):286–91.

Dhurat R, Sukesh M. Principles and methods of preparation of platelet-rich plasma: a review and author's perspective. J Cutan Aesthet Surg. 2014;7(4):189–97.

Diefenbach GJ, Tolin DF, Crocetto JS, Maltby N, Hannan SE. Assessment of trichotillomania: A psychometric evaluation of hair-pulling scales. *J Psychopathol Behav Assess.* 2005;27:169–78.

Dillon KL. A comprehensive literature review of JAK inhibitors in treatment of alopecia areata. *Clin Cosmet Investig Dermatol.* 2021;14:691–714.

Dlova NC, Salkey KS, Callender VD, McMichael AJ. Central centrifugal cicatricial alopecia: New insights and a call for action. *J Investig Dermatol Symp Proc.* 2017;18(2):S54–6.

Dowd M, Antonov N, Garzon M, Lauren C. Successful use of topical minoxidil in the treatment of hypotrichosis associated with desmoplakin mutations. *Pediatr Dermatol.* 2019;36(6):1010–11.

Drake L, Reyes-Hadsall S, Martinez J, Heinrich C, Huang K, Mostaghimi A. Evaluation of the safety and effectiveness of nutritional supplements for treating hair loss: A systematic review. *JAMA Dermatol.* 2023;159(1):79–86.

Duvic M, Lemak NA, Valero V, Hymes SR, Farmer KL, Hortobagyi GN, Trancik RJ, Bandstra BA, Compton LD. A randomized trial of minoxidil in chemotherapy-induced alopecia. *J Am Acad Dermatol.* 1996;35(1):74–8.

Dy L. A single-center study evaluating Alma TED™ and a peptide-based topical hair care formula for a variety of hair loss concerns [internet], Alma Lasers, 2023. https://californiahairsurgeon.com/wp-content/uploads/Alma-TED-Dy-Whitepaper-FIN2.pdf.

Earles RM. Surgical correction of traumatic alopecia marginalis or traction alopecia in Black women. *J Dermatol Surg Oncol.* 1986;12(1):78–82.

El-Mosallamy AE, Sleem AA, Abdel-Salam OM, Shaffie N, Kenawy SA. Antihypertensive and cardioprotective effects of pumpkin seed oil. *J Med Food.* 2012;15(2):180–9.

El Sayed MH, Abdallah MA, Aly DG, Khater NH. Association of metabolic syndrome with female pattern hair loss in women: a case-control study. Int J Dermatol. 2016;55(10):1131–7.

El-Taweel AE, El-Esawy F, Abdel-Salam O. Different trichoscopic features of tinea capitis and alopecia areata in pediatric patients. *Dermatol Res Pract.* 2014;2014:848763.

Elena EP, Irina OS. Combination therapy with platelet-rich plasma and minoxidil leads to better clinical results than monotherapy with these methods in men with androgenetic alopecia. *Int J Trichology.* 2022;14(1):1–7.

Elghblawi E. Idiosyncratic findings in trichoscopy of tinea capitis: Comma, zigzag hairs, corkscrew, and morse code-like hair. *Int J Trichol.* 2016;8(4):180–3.

Elmaadawi IH, Mohamed BM, Ibrahim ZAS, Abdou SM, El Attar YA, Youssef A, Salem ML. Stem cell therapy as a novel therapeutic intervention for resistant cases of alopecia areata and androgenetic alopecia. *J Dermatol Treat.* 2018;29(5):431–40.

Endo Y, Obayashi Y, Ono T, Serizawa T, Murakoshi M, Ohyama M. Reversal of the hair loss phenotype by modulating the estradiol-ANGPT2 axis in the mouse model of female pattern hair loss. *J Dermatol Sci.* 2018;91(1):43–51.

Erdemir F, Harbin A, Hellstrom WJ. 5-alpha reductase inhibitors and erectile dysfunction: The connection. *J Sex Med.* 2008;5(12):2917–24.

Ersan M, Ozer E, Akin O, Tasli PN, Sahin F. Effectiveness of exosome treatment in androgenetic alopecia: Outcomes of a prospective study. *Aesthetic Plast Surg.* 2024;48(21):4262–71.

Esfandiari A, Kelly AP. The effects of tea polyphenolic compounds on hair loss among rodents. *J Natl Med Assoc.* 2005;97(8):1165–9.

Esmat SM, Hegazy RA, Gawdat HI, Abdel Hay RM, Allam RS, El Naggar R, et al. Low level light–minoxidil 5% combination versus either therapeutic modality alone in management of female-patterned hair loss: a randomized controlled study. *Lasers Surg Med.* 2017;49(9):835–43.

Etzioni RD, Howlader N, Shaw PA, Ankerst DP, Penson DF, Goodman PJ, Thompson IM. Long-term effects of finasteride on prostate-specific antigen levels: Results from the prostate cancer prevention trial. *J Urol.* 2005;174(3):877–81. Erratum in: *J Urol.* 2005;174(5):2071.

Eun HC, Kwon OS, Yeon JH, Shin HS, Kim BY, Ro BI, et al. Efficacy, safety, and tolerability of dutasteride 0.5 mg once daily in male patients with male pattern hair loss: A randomized, double-blind, placebo-controlled, phase III study. *J Am Acad Dermatol.* 2010;63(2):252–8.

Evron E, Juhasz M, Babadjouni A, Mesinkovska NA. Natural hair supplement: Friend or foe? Saw palmetto, a systematic review in alopecia. *Skin Appendage Disord.* 2020;6(6):329–37.

Fabbrocini G, Cantelli M, Masarà A, Annunziata MC, Marasca C, Cacciapuoti S. Female pattern hair loss: a clinical, pathophysiologic, and therapeutic review. *Int J Womens Dermatol.* 2018;4(4):203–11.

Faden DF, Xie L, Stone C, Lopes Almeida Gomes L, Le T, Ezeh N, Buckingham WR, Kind A, Vleugels RA, Werth VP, Arkin L, Shaw KS. Area deprivation and disease severity in adult patients with discoid lupus erythematosus. *JAMA Dermatol.* 2024;160(9):984–8.

Fang Q, Chen P, Du N, Nandakumar KS. Analysis of data from breast diseases treated with 5-alpha reductase inhibitors for benign prostatic hyperplasia. *Clin Breast Cancer.* 2019;19(5):e624–36.

Farkas HS, Jee YH, Szymczuk V, Leschek EW. Persistent gynecomastia due to short-term low-dose finasteride for androgenetic alopecia. *JCEM Case Rep.* 2024;2(5):luae050.

Fertig RM, Gamret AC, Cervantes J, Tosti A. Microneedling for the treatment of hair loss? *J Eur Acad Dermatol Venereol.* 2018;32(4):564–9.

Fields JR, Vonu PM, Monir RL, Schoch JJ. Topical ketoconazole for the treatment of androgenetic alopecia: A systematic review. *Dermatol Ther.* 2020;33(1):e13202.

Fischer TW, Burmeister G, Schmidt HW, Elsner P. Melatonin increases anagen hair rate in women with androgenetic alopecia or diffuse alopecia: Results of a pilot randomized controlled trial. *Br J Dermatol.* 2004 Feb;150(2):341–5.

Fischer TW, Hipler UC, Elsner P. Effect of caffeine and testosterone on the proliferation of human hair follicles in vitro. *Int J Dermatol.* 2007;46(1):27–35.

Fischer TW, Slominski A, Tobin DJ, Paus R. Melatonin and the hair follicle. *J Pineal Res.* 2008;44(1):1–15.

Fischer TW, Trüeb RM, Hänggi G, Innocenti M, Elsner P. Topical melatonin for treatment of androgenetic alopecia. *Int J Trichology.* 2012;4(4):236–45.

Foster KW, Friedlander SF, Panzer H, Ghannoum MA, Elewski BE. A randomized controlled trial assessing the efficacy of fluconazole in the treatment of pediatric tinea capitis. *J Am Acad Dermatol.* 2005;53(5):798–809.

Fransway AF, Fransway PJ, Belsito DV, Yiannias JA. Paraben toxicology. *Dermatitis.* 2019;30(1):32–45.

Freire PCB, Riera R, Martimbianco ALC, Petri V, Atallah AN. Minoxidil for patchy alopecia areata: Systematic review and meta-analysis. *J Eur Acad Dermatol Venereol.* 2019;33(9):1792–9.

Friedlander SF, Aly R, Krafchik B, Blumer J, Honig P, Stewart D, et al. Tinea Capitis study group. Terbinafine in the treatment of *Trichophyton* tinea capitis: A randomized, double-blind, parallel-group, duration-finding study. *Pediatrics.* 2002;109(4):602–7.

Fukuoka H, Suga H. Hair regeneration treatment using adipose-derived stem cell conditioned medium: Follow-up with trichograms. *Eplasty.* 2015;15:e10.

Fuller LC, Barton RC, Mohd Mustapa MF, Proudfoot LE, Punjabi SP, Higgins EM. British Association of Dermatologists' guidelines for the management of tinea capitis 2014. *Br J Dermatol.* 2014;171(3):454–63.

Galior K, Grebe S, Singh R. Development of vitamin D toxicity from overcorrection of vitamin D deficiency: A review of case reports. *Nutrients.* 2018;10(8):953.

Gan Y, Du L, Wang H, Li K, Fan Z, Sun P, Zhang J, Hu Z, Miao Y. A clinical trial of treating androgenic alopecia with mesenchymal stem cell suspension derived from autologous hair follicle. *Plast Reconstr Surg.* 2024;154(3):444e–50e.

Garg S, Manchanda S. Platelet-rich plasma-an 'Elixir' for treatment of alopecia: personal experience on 117 patients with review of literature. *Stem Cell Investig.* 2017;Jul18;4:64. doi: 10.21037/sci.2017.06.07.

Gasteratos K, Kouzounis K, Goverman J. Autologous stem cell-derived therapies for androgenetic alopecia: A systematic review of randomized control trials on efficacy, safety, and outcomes. *Plast Reconstr Surg Glob Open.* 2024;12(2):e5606.

Gentile P, Garcovich S. Advances in regenerative stem cell therapy in androgenic alopecia and hair loss: Wnt pathway, growth-factor, and mesenchymal stem cell signaling impact analysis on cell growth and hair follicle development. *Cells.* 2019;8(5):466.

Gentile P, Garcovich S, Bielli A, Scioli MG, Orlandi A, Cervelli V. The effect of platelet-rich plasma in hair regrowth: a randomized placebo-controlled trial. *Stem Cells Transl Med.* 2015;4(11):1317–23.

Gentile P, Garcovich S, Perego F, Arsiwala N, Yavuz MF, Pessei V, Pusceddu T, Zavan B, Arsiwala S. Autologous micrografts containing nanovesicles, exosomes, and follicle stem cells in androgenetic alopecia: In vitro and in vivo analysis through a multicentric, observational, evaluator-blinded study. *Aesthet Plast Surg.* 2024;49(1):43–58.

Georgala S, Katoulis AC, Befon A. Topical estrogen therapy for androgenetic alopecia in menopausal females. *Dermatology.* 2004;208(2):178–9.

Gerkowicz A, Chyl-Surdacka K, Krasowska D, Chodorowska G. The role of vitamin D in non-scarring alopecia. *Int J Mol Sci.* 2017;18(12):2653.

Giordano S, Romeo M, Lankinen P. Platelet-rich plasma for androgenetic alopecia: does it work? Evidence from meta-analysis. *J Cosmet Dermatol.* 2017;16(3):374–81.

Gisleskog PO, Hermann D, Hammarlund-Udenaes M, Karlsson MO. The pharmacokinetic modeling of GI198745 (dutasteride), a compound with parallel linear and nonlinear elimination. *Br J Clin Pharmacol.* 1999;47(1):53–8.

Goepel M, Hecker U, Krege S, Rübben H, Michel MC. Saw palmetto extracts potently and noncompetitively inhibit human α1-adrenoceptors in vitro. *Prostate.* 1999;38(3):208–15.

Gokce N, Basgoz N, Kenanoglu S, Akalin H, Ozkul Y, Ergoren MC, Beccari T, Bertelli M, Dundar M. An overview of the genetic aspects of hair loss and its connection with nutrition. *J Prev Med Hyg.* 2022;63(2 Suppl 3):E228–38.

Goren A, Sharma A, Dhurat R, Shapiro J, Sinclair R, Situm M, Kovacevic M, Lukinovic Skudar V, Goldust M, Lotti T, McCoy J. Low-dose daily aspirin reduces topical minoxidil efficacy in androgenetic alopecia patients. *Dermatol Ther.* 2018;31(6):e12741.

Gossell-Williams M, Davis A, O'Connor N. Inhibition of testosterone-induced hyperplasia of the prostate of Sprague-Dawley rats by pumpkin seed oil. *J Med Food.* 2006;9(2):284–6.

Gowda SK, Errichetti E, Thakur V, Panda M, Dash S, Agarwal A, Sethy M, Ayyanar P, Behera B. Trichoscopic features of scalp discoid lupus erythematosus versus lichen planopilaris: A systematic review. *Clin Cosmet Investig Dermatol.* 2024;17:805–27.

Grant JE, Dougherty DD, Chamberlain SR. Prevalence, gender correlates, and co-morbidity of trichotillomania. *Psychiatry Res.* 2020;288:112948.

Greer DL. Successful treatment of tinea capitis with 2% ketoconazole shampoo. *Int J Dermatol.* 2000 Apr;39(4):302–4.

Grover C, Khurana A. Telogen effluvium. *Indian J Dermatol Venereol Leprol.* 2013;79:591–603.

Grymowicz M, Rudnicka E, Podfigurna A, Napierala P, Smolarczyk R, Smolarczyk K, Meczekalski B. Hormonal effects on hair follicles. *Int J Mol Sci.* 2020;21(15):5342.

Gubelin Harcha W, Barboza Martínez J, Tsai TF, Katsuoka K, Kawashima M, Tsuboi R, Barnes A, Ferron-Brady G, Chetty D. A randomized, active- and placebo-controlled study of the efficacy and safety of different doses of dutasteride versus placebo and finasteride in the treatment of male subjects with androgenetic alopecia. *J Am Acad Dermatol.* 2014;70(3):489–98.e3.

Guess HA, Gormley GJ, Stoner E, Oesterling JE. The effect of finasteride on prostate-specific antigen: Review of available data. *J Urol.* 1996;155(1):3–9.

Gupta AK, Adam P, Dlova N, Lynde CW, Hofstader S, Morar N, et al. Therapeutic options for the treatment of tinea capitis caused by *Trichophyton* species: Griseofulvin versus the new oral antifungal agents, terbinafine, itraconazole, and fluconazole. *Pediatr Dermatol.* 2001;18(5):433–8.

Gupta AK, Drummond-Main C. Meta-analysis of randomized, controlled trials comparing particular doses of griseofulvin and terbinafine for the treatment of tinea capitis. *Pediatr Dermatol.* 2013;30(1):1–6.

Gupta AK, Mays RR, Versteeg SG, Piraccini BM, Shear NH, Piguet V, et al. Tinea capitis in children: A systematic review of management. *J Eur Acad Dermatol Venereol.* 2018;32(12):2264–74.

Gupta M, Mahajan VK, Mehta KS, Chauhan PS. Zinc therapy in dermatology: a review. *Dermatol Res Pract.* 2014;2014:709152.

Gupta M, Mysore V. Classifications of patterned hair loss: a review. J Cutan Aesthet Surg. 2016;9(1):3–12.

Gupta AK, Quinlan EM, Venkataraman M, Bamimore MA. Microneedling for hair loss. *J Cosmet Dermatol.* 2022;21(1):108–17.

Gupta AK, Wang T, Rapaport JA. Systematic review of exosome treatment in hair restoration: Preliminary evidence, safety, and future directions. *J Cosmet Dermatol.* 2023;22(9):2424–33.

Gupta AK, Wang T, Vincent K, Abramovits W. Olumiant® (Baricitinib)-A newly approved Janus kinase inhibitor for the treatment of alopecia areata. *Skinmed.* 2022;20(6):452–55.

Hamblin MR. Mechanisms and applications of the anti-inflammatory effects of photobiomodulation. *AIMS Biophys.* 2017;4(3):337–61.

Haroon TS, Hussain I, Aman S, Jahangir M, Kazmi AH, Sami AR, et al. A randomized double-blind comparative study of terbinafine for 1, 2, and 4 weeks in tinea capitis. *Br J Dermatol.* 1996 Jul;135(1):86–8.

Haroon TS, Hussain I, Aman S, Jahangir M, Kazmi AH, Sami AR, et al. Randomized double-blind multicentre study of efficacy and tolerability of terbinafine for 1, 2, and 4 weeks in the treatment of tinea capitis. *J Eur Acad Dermatol Venereol.* 1995;5(Suppl 1):s79–80.

Harrison S, Bergfeld W. Diffuse hair loss: Its triggers and management. *Cleve Clin J Med.* 2009;76:361–7.

Hassan L, Samin KA, Mohsin S, Asif MI, Maheshwary N, Ahmed A. Compare the efficacy of PRP intervention vs exosomes for hair loss: a case series study. *Dermatol Pract Res.* 2024;4(3). doi:10.35702/Derm.10019.

He Y, Liu X, Qu Q, Chen J, Fan Z, Zhu D, Miao Y, Hu Z. Overexpression of miR-122 promotes apoptosis of dermal papilla cells by directly targeting IGF1R in androgenetic alopecia. *Cell Biol Int.* 2022;46(2):185–91.

Heath CR, Taylor SC. Alopecia in an ophiasis pattern: Traction alopecia versus alopecia areata. *Cutis.* 2012;89(5):213-6.

Heilmann-Heimbach S, Herold C, Hochfeld LM, Hillmer AM, Nyholt DR, Hecker J. Meta-analysis identifies novel risk loci and yields systematic insights into the biology of male-pattern baldness. *Nat Commun.* 2017;8:1–12.

Herskovitz I, Miteva M. Central centrifugal cicatricial alopecia: Challenges and solutions. *Clin Cosmet Investig Dermatol.* 2016;9:175–81.

Herskovitz I, Tosti A. Female pattern hair loss. *Int J Endocrinol Metab.* 2013;11(4):e9860.

Herz-Ruelas ME, Álvarez-Villalobos NA, Millán-Alanís JM, de León-Gutiérrez H, Ocampo-Garza SS, Gómez-Flores M, Grimalt R. Efficacy of intralesional and oral dutasteride in the treatment of androgenetic alopecia: A systematic review. *Skin Appendage Disord.* 2020;6(6):338–45.

Higgins CA, Christiano AM. Regenerative medicine and hair loss: How hair follicle culture has advanced our understanding of treatment options for androgenetic alopecia. *Regen Med.* 2014;9(1):101–11.

Hirshburg JM, Kelsey PA, Therrien CA, Gavino AC, Reichenberg JS. Adverse effects and safety of 5-alpha reductase inhibitors (finasteride, dutasteride): A systematic review. *J Clin Aesthet Dermatol.* 2016;9(7):56–62.

Hom E. Stress and the hair growth cycle: Cortisol-induced hair growth disruption. *J Drugs Dermatol.* 2016;15(8):1001–4.

Hu S, Zhang J, Ji Q, Xie S, Jiang J, Ni H, He X, Yang Y, Wu M. Exosomes derived from uMSCs promote hair regrowth in alopecia areata through accelerating human hair follicular keratinocyte proliferation and migration. *Cell Biol Int.* 2024;48(2):154–61.

Huang B, Kang BG, Lim SS, Zhang XH. *Melandrium firmum* extract promotes hair growth by modulating 5α-reductase activity and gene expression in C57BL/6J mice. *Ann Dermatol.* 2019;31(5):502–10.
Huang SS, Zheng RL. Biphasic regulation of angiogenesis by reactive oxygen species. *Pharmazie.* 2006 Mar;61(3):223–9.
Hubbard TW. The predictive value of symptoms in diagnosing childhood tinea capitis. *Arch Pediatr Adolesc Med.* 1999;153(11):1150.
Hugo Perez BS. Ketocazole as an adjunct to finasteride in the treatment of androgenetic alopecia in men. *Med Hypotheses.* 2004;62(1):112–15.
Hwang SM, Lee WS, Choi EH, Lee SH, Ahn SK. Nurse's cap alopecia. *Int J Dermatol.* 1999;38(3):187–91.
Hwang HW, Ryou S, Jeong JH, Lee JW, Lee KJ, Lee SB, et al. The quality of life and psychosocial impact on female pattern hair loss. Ann Dermatol. 2024;36(1):44–52.
Iamsumang W, Leerunyakul K, Suchonwanit P. Finasteride and its potential for the treatment of female-pattern hair loss: Evidence to date. *Drug Des Devel Ther.* 2020 Mar 2;14:951–9.
Ibrahim IM, Hasan MS, Elsabaa KI, Elsaie ML. Pumpkin seed oil vs. minoxidil 5% topical foam for the treatment of female pattern hair loss: A randomized comparative trial. *J Cosmet Dermatol.* 2021;20(9):2867–73.
Inamadar AC. Covid-induced telogen effluvium (CITE): An insight. *Indian Dermatol Online J.* 2022 Jun 24;13(4):445–8.
Iorizzo M, Waśkiel-Burnat A, Anedda J, Piraccini BM, Apalla Z, Rudnicka L, Starace M. Persistent chemotherapy-induced alopecia treated with low-dose oral minoxidil: A multicenter retrospective case series of 15 patients. *Dermatol Pract Concept.* 2023;13(3):e2023152.
Irwig MS. Depressive symptoms and suicidal thoughts among former users of finasteride with persistent sexual side effects. *J Clin Psychiatry.* 2012;73(9):1220–3.
Ito N, Ito T, Kromminga A, Bettermann A, Takigawa M, Kees F, Straub RH, Paus R. Human hair follicles display a functional equivalent of the hypothalamic-pituitary-adrenal axis and synthesize cortisol. *FASEB J.* 2005;19(10):1332–4.
Jabbari A, Sansarcq F, Cerise J, et al. An open-label pilot study to evaluate the efficacy of tofacitinib in moderate to severe patch-type alopecia areata, totalis, and universalis. *J Invest Dermatol.* 2018;138(7):1539–45.
Jean-Pierre P, Pulumati A, Kasheri E, Hirsch M, Nouri K. Lasers in the management of alopecia: A review of established therapies and advances in treatment. *Lasers Med Sci.* 2024;39(1):102.
Jimenez JJ, Wikramanayake TC, Bergfeld W, Hordinsky M, Hickman JG, Hamblin MR, et al. Efficacy and safety of a low-level laser device in the treatment of male and female pattern hair loss: a multicenter, randomized, sham device-controlled, double-blind study. *Am J Clin Dermatol.* 2014;15(2):115–27.
Jimenez-Cauhe J, Saceda-Corralo D, Rodrigues-Barata R, Hermosa-Gelbard A, Moreno-Arrones OM, Fernandez-Nieto D, Vaño-Galvan S. Effectiveness and safety of low-dose oral minoxidil in male androgenetic alopecia. *J Am Acad Dermatol.* 2019;81(2):648–9.
Joseph AK, Windsor B, Hynan LS, Chong BF. Discoid lupus erythematosus skin lesion distribution and characteristics in Black patients: A retrospective cohort study. *Lupus Sci Med.* 2021;8(1):e000514.
Kanayama K, Kato H, Mori M, Sakae Y, Okazaki M. Robotically assisted recipient site preparation in hair restoration surgery: Surgical safety and clinical outcomes in 31 consecutive patients. *Dermatol Surg.* 2021;47(10):1365–70.
Kang BY, Li AW, Lee MH, Wong CC, Naseer N, Ibrahim SA, Miller CH, Keimig EL, Poon E, Alam M. The safety and efficacy of autologous adipose-derived stromal vascular fraction for nonscarring alopecia: A systematic review. *Arch Dermatol Res.* 2022;314(4):349–56.
Kang D, Liu Z, Qian C, Huang J, Zhou Y, Mao X, Qu Q, Liu B, Wang J, Hu Z, Miao Y. 3D bio-printing of a gelatin-alginate hydrogel for tissue-engineered hair follicle regeneration. *Acta Biomater.* 2023;165:19–30.
Kang H, Alzolibani AA, Otberg N, Shapiro J. Lichen planopilaris. *Dermatol Ther.* 2008 Jul-Aug;21(4):249–56.
Kassimir JJ. Use of topical minoxidil as a possible adjunct to hair transplant surgery: A pilot study. *J Am Acad Dermatol.* 1987;16(3 Pt 2):685–7.
Karashima T, Tsuruta D, Hamada T, Ono F, Ishii N, Abe T, et al. Oral zinc therapy for zinc deficiency-related telogen effluvium. *Dermatol Ther.* 2012;25(2):210–3.

Katz HI, Waalen J, Leach EE. Acitretin in psoriasis: An overview of adverse effects. *J Am Acad Dermatol.* 1999;41(3 Pt 2):S7–12.

Kaufman KD. Androgens and alopecia. *Mol Cell Endocrinol.* 2002;198(1–2):89–95.

Kaufman KD, Olsen EA, Whiting D, Savin R, DeVillez R, Bergfeld W, et al. Finasteride in the treatment of men with androgenetic alopecia. *J Am Acad Dermatol.* 1998;39(4 Pt 1):578–89.

Keene S, Goren A. Therapeutic hotline. Genetic variations in the androgen receptor gene and finasteride response in women with androgenetic alopecia mediated by epigenetics. *Dermatol Ther.* 2011;24(2):296–300.

Kerstein RL, Lister T, Cole R. Laser therapy and photosensitive medication: A review of the evidence. *Lasers Med Sci.* 2014;29(4):1449–52.

Khumalo N, Jessop S, Gumedze F, Ehrlich R. Hairdressing and the prevalence of scalp disease in African adults. *Br J Dermatol.* 2007;157(5):981–8.

Khumalo N, Ngwanya R. Traction alopecia: 2% topical minoxidil shows promise. Report of two cases. *J Eur Acad Dermatol Venereol.* 2007;21(3):433–4.

Khumalo NP. The “fringe sign” for public education on traction alopecia. *Dermatol Online J.* 2012;18(9):16.

Kim H, Choi JW, Kim JY, Shin JW, Lee SJ, Huh CH. Low-level light therapy for androgenetic alopecia: a 24-week, randomized, double-blind, sham device-controlled multicenter trial. *Dermatol Surg.* 2013;39(8):1177–83.

Kim JE, Lee YJ, Lee KJ, Park SH, Kang H. Ex vivo treatment with allogenic mesenchymal stem cells of a healthy donor on peripheral blood mononuclear cells of patients with severe alopecia areata: Targeting dysregulated T cells and the acquisition of immunotolerance. *Int J Mol Sci.* 2022;23(21):13228.

Kim SJ, Kim MJ, Lee YJ, Lee JC, Kim JH, Kim DH, Do YH, Choi JW, Chung SI, Do BR. Innovative method of alopecia treatment by autologous adipose-derived SVF. *Stem Cell Res Ther.* 2021;12(1):486.

Kim WS, Lee HI, Lee JW, Lim YY, Lee SJ, Kim BJ, Kim MN, Song KY, Park WS. Fractional photothermolysis laser treatment of male pattern hair loss. *Dermatol Surg.* 2011;37(1):41–51.

King B, Ohyama M, Kwon O, Zlotogorski A, Ko J, Mesinkovska NA, Hordinsky M, Dutronc Y, Wu WS, McCollam J, Chiasserini C, Yu G, Stanley S, Holzwarth K, DeLozier AM, Sinclair R, BRAVE-AA Investigators. Two phase 3 trials of baricitinib for alopecia areata. *N Engl J Med.* 2022 May 5;386(18):1687–99.

King B, Zhang X, Harcha WG, Szepietowski JC, Shapiro J, Lynde C, Mesinkovska NA, Zwillich SH, Napatalung L, Wajsbrot D, Fayyad R, Freyman A, Mitra D, Purohit V, Sinclair R, Wolk R. Efficacy and safety of ritlecitinib in adults and adolescents with alopecia areata: A randomised, double-blind, multicentre, phase 2b-3 trial. *Lancet.* 2023;401(10387):1518–29. Erratum in: *Lancet.* 2023;401(10392):1928.

Kligman AM. Pathologic dynamics of human hair loss: I. Telogen effluvium. *Arch Dermatol.* 1961;83:175–98.

Kost Y, Muskat A, Mhaimeed N, Nazarian RS, Kobets K. Exosome therapy in hair regeneration: A literature review of the evidence, challenges, and future opportunities. *J Cosmet Dermatol.* 2022;21(8):3226–31.

Kuijper EAM, Ket JC, Caanen MR, Lambalk CB. Reproductive hormone concentrations in pregnancy and neonates: A systematic review. *Reprod Biomed Online.* 2013;27(1):33–63.

Kwack MH, Ben Hamida O, Kim MK, Kim JC, Sung YK. Dexamethasone, a synthetic glucocorticoid, induces the activity of androgen receptor in human dermal papilla cells. *Skin Pharmacol Physiol.* 2022;35(5):299–304.

Kwack MH, Seo CH, Gangadaran P, Ahn BC, Kim MK, Kim JC, Sung YK. Exosomes derived from human dermal papilla cells promote hair growth in cultured human hair follicles and augment the hair-inductive capacity of cultured dermal papilla spheres. *Exp Dermatol.* 2019;28(7):854–7.

Lawson CN, Hollinger J, Sethi S, et al. Updates in the understanding and treatments of skin & hair disorders in women of color. *Int J Womens Dermatol.* 2017;3(1):S21–37.

Lee E, Choi MS, Cho BS, Won YJ, Lee JH, Kim SR, Kim MH, Jeon JH, Park GH, Kwon HH, Lee J, Park KY, Park BC. The efficacy of adipose stem cell-derived exosomes in hair regeneration based on a preclinical and clinical study. *Int J Dermatol.* 2024;63(9):1212–20.

Lee GY, Lee SJ, Kim WS. The effect of a 1550 nm fractional erbium-glass laser in female pattern hair loss. *J Eur Acad Dermatol Venereol.* 2011;25(12):1450–4.

Lee SE, Lee EY, Kang SJ, Lee SH. 11β-Hydroxysteroid dehydrogenase type 1 inhibition attenuates the adverse effects of glucocorticoids on dermal papilla cells. *Yonsei Med J.* 2017;58(6):1204–10.

Lee SW, Juhasz M, Mobasher P, Ekelem C, Mesinkovska NA. A systematic review of topical finasteride in the treatment of androgenetic alopecia in men and women. *J Drugs Dermatol.* 2018;17(4):457–63.

Lepe K, Nassereddin A, Syed HA, Salazar FJ. Lichen planopilaris. 2024 May 1. In: *StatPearls* [Internet]. Treasure Island (FL): StatPearls Publishing; 2024. https://www.ncbi.nlm.nih.gov/books/NBK470325/.

Leung AKC, Hon KL, Leong KF, Barankin B, Lam JM. Tinea capitis: An updated review. *Recent Pat Inflamm Allergy Drug Discov.* 2020;14(1):58–68.

Li D, Ferguson A, Cervinski MA, Lynch KL, Kyle PB. AACC guidance document on biotin interference in laboratory tests. *J Appl Lab Med.* 2020;5(3):575–87.

Li H, Li B. PRP as a new approach to prevent infection: Preparation and in vitro antimicrobial properties of PRP. *J Vis Exp.* 2013;(74):50351.

Li J, Zhao B, Yao S, Dai Y, Zhang X, Yang N, Bao Z, Cai J, Chen Y, Wu X. Dermal papilla cell-derived exosomes regulate hair follicle stem cell proliferation via LEF1. *Int J Mol Sci.* 2023;24(4):3961.

Li Y, Wang G, Wang Q, Zhang Y, Cui L, Huang X. Exosomes secreted from adipose-derived stem cells are a potential treatment agent for immune-mediated alopecia. *J Immunol Res.* 2022;2022:7471246.

Liang Y, Tang X, Zhang X, Cao C, Yu M, Wan M. Adipose mesenchymal stromal cell-derived exosomes carrying miR-122-5p antagonize the inhibitory effect of dihydrotestosterone on hair follicles by targeting the TGF-β1/SMAD3 signaling pathway. *Int J Mol Sci.* 2023;24(6):5703.

Lin BJ, Wang J, Miao Y, Liu YQ, Jiang W, Fan ZX, Darabi MA, Hu ZQ, Xing M. Cytokine-loaded layer-by-layer ultrathin matrices to deliver single dermal papilla cells for spot-by-spot hair follicle regeneration. *J Mater Chem B.* 2016;4(3):489–504.

Liu L, Craiglow B, King B. Tofacitinib 2% ointment, a topical Janus kinase inhibitor for the treatment of alopecia areata: A pilot study of 10 patients. *J Am Acad Dermatol.* 2018;78(2):403–4.

Liu Z, Huang J, Kang D, Zhou Y, Du L, Qu Q, et al. Microenvironmental reprogramming of human dermal papilla cells for hair follicle tissue engineering. *Acta Biomater.* 2023;165:31–49. doi:10.1016/j.actbio.2022.11.004. PMID: 36347448.

Lu K, Han Q, Ma Z, Yan Q, Pei Y, Shi P, Zhang J, Rong K, Ma K, Li P, Hou T. Injectable platelet-rich fibrin facilitates hair follicle regeneration by promoting human dermal papilla cell proliferation, migration, and trichogenic inductivity. *Exp Cell Res.* 2021;409(1):112888.

Lucky AW, Piacquadio DJ, Ditre CM, Dunlap F, Kantor I, Pandya AG, Savin RC, Tharp MD. A randomized, placebo-controlled trial of 5% and 2% topical minoxidil solutions in the treatment of female-pattern hair loss. *J Am Acad Dermatol.* 2004;50(4):541–53.

Lueangarun S, Panchaprateep R, Tempark T, Noppakun N. Efficacy and safety of oral minoxidil 5 mg daily during 24-week treatment in male androgenetic alopecia. *J Am Acad Dermatol.* 2015;72:AB113.

Lueangarun S, Visutjindaporn P, Parcharoen Y, Jamparuang P, Tempark T. A systematic review and meta-analysis of randomized controlled trials of United States Food and Drug Administration-approved, home-use, low-level light/laser therapy devices for pattern hair loss: Device design and technology. *J Clin Aesthet Dermatol.* 2021;14(11):E64–75.

Ly N, McClure EM, Hordinsky MK, Farah RS, Park SY. Safety and efficacy of minoxidil treatment in scarring alopecia: A scoping review. *J Drugs Dermatol.* 2024 Mar 1;23(3):146–51.

Ly NY, Fruechte S, Hordinsky MK, Sadick N, Arruda S, Farah RS. Medical and procedural treatment of androgenetic alopecia - Where are we? *J Am Acad Dermatol.* 2023;89(2S):S36–9.

Ma L, Chen C, Liu D, Huang Z, Li J, Liu H, Kin Kwok RT, Tang B, Sui B, Zhang X, Tang J, Mao X, Huang W, Shi S, Kou X. Apoptotic extracellular vesicles are metabolized regulators nurturing the skin and hair. *Bioact Mater.* 2022;19:626–41.

Malta M Jr, Corso G. Understanding the association between mental health and hair loss. *Cureus.* 2025;17(5):e84777.

Mammoto T, Jiang A, Jiang E, Mammoto A. Platelet-rich plasma extract promotes angiogenesis through the angiopoietin1–Tie2 pathway. Microvasc Res. 2013;89:15–24.

Marion T, Werbel T, Torres A. Reducing legal risks and social media issues for cosmetic surgery. *Facial Plast Surg Clin North Am.* 2023;31(2):333–40.

Marks DH, Prasad S, De Souza B, Burns LJ, Senna MM. Topical antiandrogen therapies for androgenetic alopecia and acne vulgaris. *Am J Clin Dermatol.* 2020;21(2):245–54.

Martinez-Jacobo L, Villarreal-Villarreal CD, Ortiz-López R, Ocampo-Candiani J, Rojas-Martínez A. Genetic and molecular aspects of androgenetic alopecia. *Indian J Dermatol Venereol Leprol.* 2018;84:263–8.

Matilainen VA, Mäkinen PK, Keinänen-Kiukaanniemi SM. Early onset of androgenetic alopecia associated with early severe coronary heart disease: A population-based, case-control study. *J Cardiovasc Risk.* 2001;8(3):147–51.

Meephansan J, Ungpraphakorn N, Ponnikorn S, Suchonwanit P, Poovorawan Y. Efficacy of 1,550-nm Erbium-Glass Fractional Laser Treatment and Its Effect on the Expression of Insulin-Like Growth Factor 1 and Wnt/β-Catenin in Androgenetic Alopecia. *Dermatol Surg.* 2018;44(10):1295–303.

Meinhard J, Stroux A, Lünnemann L, Vogt A, Blume-Peytavi U. Lichen planopilaris: Epidemiology and prevalence of subtypes - a retrospective analysis in 104 patients. *J Dtsch Dermatol Ges.* 2014;12(3):229–35, 229–36.

Memisoglu HR, Erboz S, Akkaya S, Akan T, Aksungur VL, Ünal I, et al. Comparative study of the efficacy and tolerability of 4 weeks of terbinafine therapy with 8 weeks of griseofulvin therapy in children with tinea capitis. *J Dermatol Treat.* 1999;10(3):189–93.

Mirmirani P. Hormonal changes in menopause: do they contribute to a 'midlife hair crisis' in women? *Br J Dermatol.* 2011;165(Suppl 3):7–11. doi:10.1111/j.1365-2133.2011.10629.x

Monselise A, Cohen DE, Wanser R, Shapiro J. What ages hair? *Int J Womens Dermatol.* 2015 Oct 9;1(4):161–6.

Morganti P, Fabrizi G, James B. Effect of gelatin-cystine and *Serenoa repens* extract on free radicals level and hair growth. *J Appl Cosmetol.* 1998;16:57–64.

Mostaghimi L. Dermatological assessment of hair pulling and skin picking. In: Grant JE, Stein DJ, Woods DW, Keuthen NJ, editors. *Trichotillomania, Skin picking, & other body-focused repetitive behaviors.* Arlington, VA: American Psychiatric Publishing; 2012.

Motosko CC, Bieber AK, Pomeranz MK, Stein JA, Martires KJ. Physiologic changes of pregnancy: A review of the literature. *Int J Womens Dermatol.* 2017;3(4):219–24.

Moussa M, Lajeunesse D, Hilal G, El Atat O, Haykal G, Serhal R, Chalhoub A, Khalil C, Alaaeddine N. Platelet-rich plasma (PRP) induces chondroprotection via increasing autophagy, anti-inflammatory markers, and decreasing apoptosis in human osteoarthritic cartilage. *Exp Cell Res.* 2017;352(1):146–56.

Murata K, Noguchi K, Kondo M, Onishi M, Watanabe N, Okamura K, Matsuda H. Promotion of hair growth by *Rosmarinus officinalis* leaf extract. *Phytother Res.* 2013;27(2):212–7.

Murugusundram S. Serenoa repens: does it have any role in the management of androgenetic alopecia? *J Cutan Aesthet Surg.* 2009;2(1):31–2.

Mutterperl RE, Diamond FB, Lowenthal DT. Long-term effects of minoxidil in the treatment of malignant hypertension in chronic renal failure. *J Clin Pharmacol.* 1976;16(10 Pt 1):498–509.

Nascimento IJB, Harries M, Barreto Rocha V, Thompson JY, Wong CH, Varkan HK, Sernizon Guimarães N, Rocha Arantes AJ, Soriano Marcolino M. Effect of oral minoxidil for alopecia: Systematic review. *Int J Trichology.* 2020;12(4):147–55.

Navarro VJ, Khan I, Björnsson E, Seeff LB, Serrano J, Hoofnagle JH. Liver injury from herbal and dietary supplements. *Hepatology.* 2017;65(1):363–73.

Navratil L, Kymplova J. Contraindications in noninvasive laser therapy: Truth and fiction. *J Clin Laser Med Surg.* 2002;20(6):341–3.

Nestor MS, Ablon G, Gade A, Han H, Fischer DL. Treatment options for androgenetic alopecia: Efficacy, side effects, compliance, financial considerations, and ethics. *J Cosmet Dermatol.* 2021;20(12):3759–81.

Nestor MS, Ablon G, Gade V, Han H, Daniels SE. Treatment options for androgenetic alopecia: Efficacy, side effects, compliance, financial considerations, and ethics. *J Cosmet Dermatol.* 2021;20(12):3759–81.

Nickel JC. Comparison of clinical trials with finasteride and dutasteride. *Rev Urol.* 2004;6(Suppl 9):S31–9.

Niu YL, Li YK, Gao CX, Li WW, Li L, Wang H, Shen W, Ge W. Melatonin promotes hair regeneration by modulating the Wnt/β-catenin signaling pathway. *Cell Prolif.* 2024 Sep;57(9):e13656.

Nohria A, Desai D, Sikora M, Mandal S, Shapiro J, Lo Sicco K. Combating "dread shed": The impact of overlapping topical and oral minoxidil on temporary hair shedding during oral minoxidil initiation. *JAAD Int.* 2024;15:220–4.

Norooznezhad AH, Yarani R, Payandeh M, Hoseinkhani Z, Mahmoudi H, Kiani S, et al. Treatment of persistent chemotherapy-induced hair loss (alopecia) with human mesenchymal stromal cells exosome enriched extracellular vesicles: a case report. *Heliyon.* 2023;9(4):e15165. doi:10.1016/j.heliyon.2023.e15165. PMID: 37095978; PMCID: PMC10121390.

Nuwayhyd R, Redler S, Heilmann S, Drichel D, Wolf S, Birch P, et al. Investigation of four novel male androgenetic alopecia susceptibility loci: No association with female pattern hair loss. *Arch Dermatol Res.* 2014;306:413–8.

Oh HA, Kwak J, Kim BJ, Jin HJ, Park WS, Choi SJ, Oh W, Um S. Migration Inhibitory Factor in Conditioned Medium from Human Umbilical Cord Blood-Derived Mesenchymal Stromal Cells Stimulates Hair Growth. *Cells.* 2020 May 28;9(6):1344. doi: 10.3390/cells9061344. PMID: 32481584; PMCID: PMC7349163.

Oh HG, Jung M, Jeong SY, Kim J, Han SD, Kim H, Lee S, Lee Y, You H, Park S, Kim EA, Kim TM, Kim S. Improvement of androgenic alopecia by extracellular vesicles secreted from hyaluronic acid-stimulated induced mesenchymal stem cells. *Stem Cell Res Ther.* 2024;15(1):287.

Oh JY, Park MA, Kim YC. Peppermint oil promotes hair growth without toxic signs. *Toxicol Res.* 2014;30(4):297–304.

Ohnemus U, Uenalan M, Inzunza J, Gustafsson J-Å, Paus R. The hair follicle as an estrogen target and source. *Endocr Rev.* 2006;27(6):677–706.

Oiwoh SO, Enitan AO, Adegbosin OT, Akinboro AO, Onayemi EO. Androgenetic alopecia: A review. *Niger Postgrad Med J.* 2024;31(2):85–92.

Olsen EA, DeLong ER, Weiner MS. Long-term follow-up of men with male pattern baldness treated with topical minoxidil. *J Am Acad Dermatol.* 1987;16(3 Pt 2):688–95.

Olsen EA, Dunlap FE, Funicella T, Koperski JA, Swinehart JM, Tschen EH, Trancik RJ. A randomized clinical trial of 5% topical minoxidil versus 2% topical minoxidil and placebo in the treatment of androgenetic alopecia in men. *J Am Acad Dermatol.* 2002 Sep;47(3):377–85.

Olsen EA, Hordinsky M, Whiting D, Stough D, Hobbs S, Ellis ML, et al. The importance of dual 5α-reductase inhibition in the treatment of male pattern hair loss: results of a randomized placebo-controlled study of dutasteride versus finasteride. J Am Acad Dermatol. 2006;55(6):1014–23.

Palin MF, Faguy M, LeHoux JG, Pelletier G. Inhibitory effects of *Serenoa repens* on the kinetic of pig prostatic microsomal 5α-reductase activity. *Endocrine.* 1998;9(1):65–9.

Pan HJ, Wilding G, Uno H, Inui S, Goldsmith L, Messing E, Chang C. Evaluation of RU58841 as an anti-androgen in prostate PC3 cells and a topical anti-alopecia agent in the bald scalp of stumptailed macaques. *Endocrine.* 1998;9(1):39–43.

Panahi Y, Taghizadeh M, Marzony ET, Sahebkar A. Rosemary oil vs minoxidil 2% for the treatment of androgenetic alopecia: A randomized comparative trial. *Skinmed.* 2015;13(1):15–21.

Panchaprateep R, Asawanonda P. Insulin-like growth factor-1: Roles in androgenetic alopecia. *Exp Dermatol.* 2014;23(3):216–18.

Panteleyev AA. Functional anatomy of the hair follicle: The secondary hair germ. *Exp Dermatol.* 2018;27(7):701–20.

Pappas PG, Kauffman CA, Perfect J, et al. Alopecia associated with fluconazole therapy. *Ann Intern Med.* 1995;123(5):354–7.

Park BS, Choi HI, Huh G, Kim WS. Effects of exosome from adipose-derived stem cell on hair loss: a retrospective analysis of 39 patients. *J Cosmet Dermatol.* 2022;21(6):2282–4.

Park J, Jun EK, Son D, Hong W, Jang J, Yun W, Yoon BS, Song G, Kim IY, You S. Overexpression of Nanog in amniotic fluid-derived mesenchymal stem cells accelerates dermal papilla cell activity and promotes hair follicle regeneration. *Exp Mol Med.* 2019;51(7):1–15.

Park SY, Na SY, Kim JH, Cho S, Lee JH. Iron plays a certain role in patterned hair loss. J Korean Med Sci. 2013;28(6):934–8.

Patel DP, Swink SM, Castelo-Soccio L. A review of the use of biotin for hair loss. *Skin Appendage Disord.* 2017;3(3):166–9.

Patel P, Nessel TA, Kumar DD. Minoxidil. In: *StatPearls* [Internet]. Treasure Island (FL): StatPearls Publishing; 2024. https://www.ncbi.nlm.nih.gov/books/NBK482378/.

Paus R, Cotsarelis G. The biology of hair follicles. *N Engl J Med.* 1999;341(7):491–7.

Pejcic AV, Paudel V. Alopecia associated with the use of selective serotonin reuptake inhibitors: A systematic review. *Psychiatry Res.* 2022;313:114620.

Penha MA, Miot HA, Kasprzak M, Müller Ramos P. Oral minoxidil vs topical minoxidil for male androgenetic alopecia: A randomized clinical trial. *JAMA Dermatol.* 2024;160(6):600–5.

Pereira-Silva M, Martins AM, Sousa-Oliveira I, Ribeiro HM, Veiga F, Marto J, Paiva-Santos AC. Nanomaterials in hair care and treatment. *Acta Biomater.* 2022;142:14–35.

Perera E, Sinclair R. Treatment of chronic telogen effluvium with oral minoxidil: A retrospective study. *F1000Res.* 2017;6:1650.

Philpott MP, Sanders D, Westgate GE, Kealey T. Human hair growth in vitro: A model for the study of hair follicle biology. *J Dermatol Sci.* 1994 Jul;7 Suppl:S55–72.

Pickrell JK, Berisa T, Liu JZ, Segura L, Tung JY, Hinds DA. Detection and interpretation of shared genetic influences on 42 human traits. *Nat Genet.* 2016;48:709–17.

Piérard-Franchimont C, De Doncker P, Cauwenbergh G, Piérard GE. Ketoconazole shampoo: Effect of long-term use in androgenic alopecia. *Dermatology.* 1998;196(4):474–7.

Pietrauszka K, Bergler-Czop B. Sulfotransferase SULT1A1 activity in hair follicle, a prognostic marker of response to the minoxidil treatment in patients with androgenetic alopecia: A review. *Postepy Dermatol Alergol.* 2022;39(3):472–8.

Pillai JK, Mysore V. Role of low-level light therapy (LLLT) in androgenetic alopecia. J Cutan Aesthet Surg. 2021;14(4):385–91.

Pinto A, Terskikh AV. The rise of induced pluripotent stem cell approach to hair restoration. *Plast Reconstr Surg.* 2021;148(6S):39S–46S.

Piraccini BM, Blume-Peytavi U, Scarci F, Jansat JM, Falqués M, Otero R, Tamarit ML, Galván J, Tebbs V, Massana E, Topical Finasteride Study Group. Efficacy and safety of topical finasteride spray solution for male androgenetic alopecia: A phase III, randomized, controlled clinical trial. *J Eur Acad Dermatol Venereol.* 2022;36(2):286–94.

Piraccini BM, Iorizzo M, Rech G, Tosti A. Drug-induced hair disorders. *Curr Drug Saf.* 2006;1(3):301–5.

Poblet E, Ortega F, Jiménez F. The arrector pili muscle and the follicular unit of the scalp: A microscopic anatomy study. *Dermatol Surg.* 2002;28(9):800–3.

Pomeranz AJ, Sabnis SS. Tinea capitis: Epidemiology, diagnosis, and management strategies. *Paediatr Drugs.* 2002;4(12):779–83.

Poulos GA, Brodell RT, Mostow EN. Improving quality and patient satisfaction in dermatology office practice. *Arch Dermatol.* 2008;144(2):263–5.

Prahalada S, Tarantal AF, Harris GS, Ellsworth KP, Clarke AP, Skiles GL, MacKenzie KI, Kruk LF, Ablin DS, Cukierski MA, Peter CP, vanZwieten MJ, Hendrickx AG. Effects of finasteride, a type 2 5-alpha reductase inhibitor, on fetal development in the rhesus monkey (*Macaca mulatta*). *Teratology.* 1997;55(2):119–31.

Prasad S, De Souza B, Burns LJ, Lippincott M, Senna MM. Polycystic ovary syndrome in patients with hair thinning. *J Am Acad Dermatol.* 2020;83(1):260–1.

Presley CL, Kolodziejczyk TC, Pulsipher KJ, et al. A scoping review of pharmacotherapy, complementary, and alternative medicine (CAM), and surgical therapies for androgenic alopecia. *Curr Derm Rep.* 2021;10:48–54.

Pulat S, Subedi L, Pandey P, Bhosle SR, Hur JS, Shim JH, Cho SS, Kim KT, Ha HH, Kim H, Park JW. Topical delivery of atraric acid derived from *Stereocaulon japonicum* with enhanced skin permeation and hair regrowth activity for androgenic alopecia. *Pharmaceutics.* 2023;15(2):340.

Queen D, Avram MR. Exosomes for treating hair loss: A review of clinical studies. *Dermatol Surg.* 2024;51(4):409–15.

Rabe T, Kowald A, Ortmann J, Rehberger-Schneider S. Inhibition of skin 5 alpha-reductase by oral contraceptive progestins in vitro. *Gynecol Endocrinol.* 2000;14(4):223–0.

Rahmani W, Sinha S, Biernaskie J. Immune modulation of hair follicle regeneration. *NPJ Regen Med.* 2020;5:9.

Ramos PM, Gohad P, McCoy J, Wambier C, Goren A. Minoxidil Sulfotransferase Enzyme (SULT1A1) genetic variants predict response to oral minoxidil treatment for female pattern hair loss. *J Eur Acad Dermatol Venereol.* 2021;35(1):e24–6.

Ramos PM, Miot HA. Female pattern hair loss: A clinical and pathophysiological review. *An Bras Dermatol.* 2015;90(4):529–43.

Randolph M, Tosti A. Oral minoxidil treatment for hair loss: A review of efficacy and safety. *J Am Acad Dermatol.* 2021;84(3):737–46.

Raposo G, Stoorvogel W. Extracellular vesicles: Exosomes, microvesicles, and friends. *J Cell Biol.* 2013;200(4):373–83.

Rassman WR, Pak JP, Kim J, Estrin NF. Scalp micropigmentation: A concealer for hair and scalp deformities. *J Clin Aesthet Dermatol.* 2015;8(3):35–42.

Rathnayake D, Sinclair R. Male androgenetic alopecia. *Expert Opin Pharmacother.* 2010;11(8):1295–304.

Raval RS, Nohria A, Desai D, Mourtzanakis K, Buontempo M, Shapiro J, Lo Sicco K. The use of minoxidil in the treatment of alopecia areata: A systematic review. *J Am Acad Dermatol.* 2024;91(3):508–9.

Raynaud JP, Cousse H, Martin PM. Inhibition of type 1 and type 2 5α-reductase activity by free fatty acids, active ingredients of Permixon. *J Steroid Biochem Mol Biol.* 2002 Oct;82(2–3):233–9.

Rebora A. Telogen effluvium: A comprehensive review. *Clin Cosmet Investig Dermatol.* 2019;12:583–90.

Redler S, Messenger AG, Betz RC. Genetics and other factors in the aetiology of female pattern hair loss. *Exp Dermatol.* 2017;26(6):510–7.

Redman MW, Tangen CM, Goodman PJ, Lucia MS, Coltman CA Jr, Thompson IM. Finasteride does not increase the risk of high-grade prostate cancer: A bias-adjusted modeling approach. *Cancer Prev Res (Phila).* 2008;1:174–81.

Reynolds RV, Yeung H, Cheng CE, Cook-Bolden F, Desai SR, Druby KM, Freeman EE, Keri JE, Stein Gold LF, Tan JKL, Tollefson MM, Weiss JS, Wu PA, Zaenglein AL, Han JM, Barbieri JS. Guidelines of care for the management of acne vulgaris. *J Am Acad Dermatol.* 2024;90(5):1006.e1–30.

Riedel-Baima B, Riedel A. Use of the TrichoScan to assess female pattern hair loss. *Dermatol Surg.* 2008;34(5):651–5.

Rinaldi F, Trink A, Mondadori G, Giuliani G, Pinto D. The menopausal transition: Is the hair follicle "going through menopause"? *Biomedicines.* 2023;11(11):3041.

Roberts J, Desai N, McCoy J, Goren A. Sulfotransferase activity in plucked hair follicles predicts response to topical minoxidil in the treatment of female androgenetic alopecia. *Dermatol Ther.* 2014;27(4):252–4.

Roehrborn C. Saw palmetto for benign prostatic hyperplasia: Just how effective is it? *Nat Rev Urol.* 2006;3:420–1.

Roohaninasab M, Goodarzi A, Ghassemi M, Sadeghzadeh-Bazargan A, Behrangi E, Najar Nobari N. Systematic review of platelet-rich plasma in treating alopecia: Focusing on efficacy, safety, and therapeutic durability. *Dermatol Ther.* 2021;34(2):e14768.

Rose PT, Nusbaum B. Robotic hair restoration. *Dermatol Clin.* 2014;32(1):97–107.

Rossi A, Cantisani C, Scarnò M, Trucchia A, Fortuna MC, Calvieri S. Finasteride, 1 mg daily administration on male androgenetic alopecia in different age groups: 10-year follow-up. *Dermatol Ther.* 2011;24(4):455–61.

Rossi A, Iorio A, Scali E, Fortuna MC, Mari E, Palese E, Greco P, Carlesimo M. Monilethrix treated with minoxidil. *Int J Immunopathol Pharmacol.* 2011 Jan-Mar;24(1):239–42.

Rossi A, Mari E, Scarno M, Garelli V, Maxia C, Scali E, Iorio A, Carlesimo M. Comparative effectiveness of finasteride vs *Serenoa repens* in male androgenetic alopecia: A two-year study. *Int J Immunopathol Pharmacol.* 2012;25(4):1167–73.

Rothbaum BO, Ninan PT. The assessment of trichotillomania. *Behav Res Ther.* 1994;32(6):651–62.

Rushton DH, Ramsay ID. The importance of adequate serum ferritin levels during oral cyproterone acetate and ethinyl oestradiol treatment of diffuse androgen-dependent alopecia in women. *Clin Endocrinol (Oxf).* 1992;36(4):421–7.

Saceda-Corralo D, Moustafa F, Moreno-Arrones Ó, Jaén-Olasolo P, Vañó-Galván S, Camacho F. Mesotherapy with dutasteride for androgenetic alopecia: A retrospective study in real clinical practice. *J Drugs Dermatol.* 2022;21(7):742–7.

Salah M, Samy N, Fawzy MM, Farrag AR, Shehata H, Hany A. The effect of the fractional carbon dioxide laser on improving minoxidil delivery for the treatment of androgenetic alopecia. *J Lasers Med Sci.* 2020;11(1):29–36.

Salazar E, Asz-Sigall D, Vega D, Arenas R. Tinea capitis: Unusual chronic presentation in an elderly woman. *J Infect Dis Epidemiol.* 2018;4:048.

Sánchez-Meza E, Ocampo-Candiani J, Gómez-Flores M, Herz-Ruelas ME, Ocampo-Garza J, Orizaga-Y-Quiroga TL, Martínez-Moreno A, Ocampo-Garza SS. Microneedling plus topical dutasteride solution for androgenetic alopecia: A randomized placebo-controlled study. *J Eur Acad Dermatol Venereol.* 2022;36(10):e806–8.

Sarkar R, Kaur H, Mendiratta V. Transient hair loss of infancy. Asian J Pediatr Dermatol. 2024;2(2):75–6.

Sattar F, Almas U, Ibrahim NA, Akhtar A, Shazad MK, Akram S, Khan MSN, Murtaza G. Efficacy of oral vitamin D3 therapy in patients suffering from diffuse hair loss (Telogen Effluvium). *J Nutr Sci Vitaminol.* 2021;67(1):68–71.

Seah BC, Teo BM. Recent advances in ultrasound-based transdermal drug delivery. *Int J Nanomedicine.* 2018;13:7749–63.

Seattle Children's. Hair loss. Accessed July 1, 2025. Available from: https://www.seattlechildrens.org/conditions/a-z/hair-loss/

Seifert B, Passweg JR, Heim D, Rovó A, Meyer-Monard S, Buechner S, Tichelli A, Gratwohl A. Complete remission of alopecia universalis after allogeneic hematopoietic stem cell transplantation. *Blood.* 2005;105(1):426–7.

Senna M, Mostaghimi A, Ohyama M, Sinclair R, Dutronc Y, Wu WS, Yu G, Chiasserini C, Somani N, Holzwarth K, King B. Long-term efficacy and safety of baricitinib in patients with severe alopecia areata: 104-week results from BRAVE-AA1 and BRAVE-AA2. *J Eur Acad Dermatol Venereol.* 2024 Mar;38(3):583–93.

Sever MS, Sonmez YE, Kocak N. Limited use of minoxidil in renal transplant recipients because of the additive side-effects of cyclosporine on hypertrichosis. Transplantation. 1990;50(3):536.

Shaban A, Sahu RP. Pumpkin seed oil: An alternative medicine. *Int J Pharmacogn Phytochem Res.* 2017;9(2):11.

Shah KB, Shah AN, Solanki RB, Raval RC. A comparative study of microneedling with platelet-rich plasma plus topical minoxidil (5%) and topical minoxidil (5%) alone in androgenetic alopecia. *Int J Trichology.* 2017;9(1):14–18.

Sharma A, Goren A, Dhurat R, Agrawal S, Sinclair R, Trüeb RM, Vañó-Galván S, Chen G, Tan Y, Kovacevic M, Situm M, McCoy J. Tretinoin enhances minoxidil response in androgenetic alopecia patients by upregulating follicular sulfotransferase enzymes. *Dermatol Ther.* 2019 May;32(3):e12915.

Sharquie KE, Jabbar RI. COVID-19 infection is a major cause of acute telogen effluvium. *Ir J Med Sci.* 2022;191(4):1677–81.

Shauly O, Marxen T, Goel P, Gould DJ. The new era of marketing in plastic surgery: A systematic review and algorithm of social media and digital marketing. *Aesthet Surg J Open Forum.* 2023;5:ojad024.

Shen Y, Sun J, Zhu Y, Chen Y, Hu Y, Luo H, Song X. Effect of fractional laser alone or in combination on alopecia areata: A systematic review and meta-analysis. *J Cosmet Dermatol.* 2023;22(5):1528–35.

Silke R, Messenger AG, Betz RC. Genetics and other factors in the aetiology of female pattern hair loss. Exp Dermatol. 2017;26:510–17.

Silva H. Current knowledge on the vascular effects of menthol. *Front Physiol.* 2020 Apr 7;11:298. https://doi.org/10.3389/fphys.2020.00298. Erratum in: *Front Physiol.* 2020;11:602231.

Sinclair R. Treatment of monilethrix with oral minoxidil. *JAAD Case Rep.* 2016;2(3):212–5.

Sinclair R, Wewerinke M, Jolley D. Treatment of female pattern hair loss with oral antiandrogens. *Br J Dermatol.* 2005;152(3):466–73.

Sinclair RD. Female pattern hair loss: A pilot study investigating combination therapy with low-dose oral minoxidil and spironolactone. *Int J Dermatol.* 2018;57(1):104–9.

Sinclair RD, Dawber RP. Androgenetic alopecia in men and women. *Clin Dermatol.* 2001;19:167–78.

Singh MK, Avram M. Persistent sexual dysfunction and depression in finasteride users for male pattern hair loss: A serious concern or red herring? *J Clin Aesthet Dermatol.* 2014;7(12):51–5.

Sintov A, Serafimovich S, Gilhar A. New topical antiandrogenic formulations can stimulate hair growth in human bald scalp grafted onto mice. *Int J Pharm.* 2000;194(1):125–34.

Slowinska M, Rudnicka L, Schwartz RA, Kowalska-Oledzka E, Rakowska A, Sicinska J, et al. Comma hairs: A dermatoscopic marker for tinea capitis: A rapid diagnostic method. *J Am Acad Dermatol.* 2008;59(5 Suppl):S77–9.

Soutou B, Rahme S, Bizdikian AJ, Skaff S, Helou J, Tomb R. Iron supplementation may improve the patient's level of satisfaction in not-low-ferritin telogen effluvium: A real-life observational study. *Indian J Dermatol.* 2024;69(2):119–22.

Sovak M, Seligson AL, Kucerova R, Bienova M, Hajduch M, Bucek M. Fluridil, a rationally designed topical agent for androgenetic alopecia: First clinical experience. *Dermatol Surg.* 2002;28(8):678–85.

Sperling LC. Hair anatomy for the clinician. *J Am Acad Dermatol.* 1991 Jul;25(1 Pt 1):1–17.

Sperling LC. Hair and systemic disease. *Dermatol Clin.* 2001;19:711–26.

Starace M, Orlando G, Alessandrini A, Piraccini BM. Female androgenetic alopecia: An update on diagnosis and management. *Am J Clin Dermatol.* 2020;21(1):69–84.

Starr RR. Too little, too late: Ineffective regulation of dietary supplements in the United States. *Am J Public Health.* 2015;105(3):478–85.

Stevens HP, Donners S, de Bruijn J. Introducing platelet-rich stroma: Platelet-rich plasma (PRP) and stromal vascular fraction (SVF) combined for the treatment of androgenetic alopecia. *Aesthet Surg J.* 2018;38(8):811–22.

Stevens J, Khetarpal S. Platelet-rich plasma for androgenetic alopecia: a review of the literature and proposed treatment protocol. *Int J Womens Dermatol.* 2018;5(1):46–51.

Stoner E. Three-year safety and efficacy data on the use of finasteride in the treatment of benign prostatic hyperplasia. *Urology.* 1994;43(3):284–92; discussion 292–4.

Suchonwanit P, Thammarucha S, Leerunyakul K. Minoxidil and its use in hair disorders: A review. *Drug Des Devel Ther.* 2019;13:2777–86.

Taki T, Tanahashi K, Takeichi T, Yoshikawa T, Murase Y, Sugiura K, Akiyama M. Association of topical minoxidil with autosomal recessive woolly hair/hypotrichosis caused by *LIPH* pathogenic variants. *JAMA Dermatol.* 2020;156(10):1030–32.

Takwale A, Agarwal S, Holmes SC, Berth-Jones J. Tinea capitis in two elderly women: Transmission at the hairdresser. *Br J Dermatol.* 2001;144(4):898–900.

Tampucci S, Paganini V, Burgalassi S, Chetoni P, Monti D. Nanostructured drug delivery systems for targeting 5-α-reductase inhibitors to the hair follicle. *Pharmaceutics.* 2022;14(2):286.

Tang X, Cao C, Liang Y, Han L, Tu B, Yu M, Wan M. Adipose-derived stem cell exosomes antagonize the inhibitory effect of dihydrotestosterone on hair follicle growth by activating Wnt/β-catenin pathway. *Stem Cells Int.* 2023;2023:5548112.

Tanz RR, Hebert AA, Esterly NB. Treating tinea capitis: Should ketoconazole replace griseofulvin? *J Pediatr.* 1988 Jun;112(6):987–91.

Tey HL, Tan AS, Chan YC. Meta-analysis of randomized, controlled trials comparing griseofulvin and terbinafine in the treatment of tinea capitis. *J Am Acad Dermatol.* 2011;64(4):663–70.

Thepphankulngarm N, Manmuan S, Hirun N, Kraisit P. Nanotechnology-driven delivery of caffeine using ultradeformable liposomes-coated hollow mesoporous silica nanoparticles for enhanced follicular delivery and treatment of androgenetic alopecia. *Int J Mol Sci.* 2024;25(22):12170.

Thom E. Stress and the hair growth cycle: Cortisol-induced hair growth disruption. *J Drugs Dermatol.* 2016;15(8):1001–4.

Thompson IM Jr, Goodman PJ, Tangen CM, Parnes HL, Minasian LM, Godley PA, Lucia MS, Ford LG. Long-term survival of participants in the prostate cancer prevention trial. *N Engl J Med.* 2013;369(7):603–10.

Thompson IM, Goodman PJ, Tangen CM, et al. The influence of finasteride on the development of prostate cancer. *N Engl J Med.* 2003;349:215–24.

Tiede S, Bohm K, Meier N, Funk W, Paus R. Endocrine controls of primary adult human stem cell biology: Thyroid hormones stimulate keratin 15 expression, apoptosis, and differentiation in human hair follicle epithelial stem cells *in situ* and *in vitro*. *Eur J Cell Biol.* 2010;89(10):769–77.

Tomita T, Goto H, Yoshida T, Tanaka K, Sumiya K, Kohda Y. Dose-dependent valproate-induced alopecia in patients with mental disorders. *Indian J Pharmacol.* 2015;47(6):690–2.

Tosti A, Piraccini BM. Androgenetic alopecia. In: Tosti A, Piraccini BM, editors. *Diagnosis and treatment of hair disorders: An evidence-based atlas.* London: Taylor & Francis Group; 2006.

Tosti A, Whiting D, Iorizzo M, Pazzaglia M, Misciali C, Vincenzi C, Micali G. The role of scalp dermoscopy in the diagnosis of alopecia areata incognita. *J Am Acad Dermatol.* 2008 Jul;59(1):64–7.

Traish AM, Melcangi RC, Bortolato M, Garcia-Segura LM, Zitzmann M. Adverse effects of 5α-reductase inhibitors: What do we know, don't know, and need to know? *Rev Endocr Metab Disord.* 2015;16(3):177–98.

Trüeb RM, Caballero-Uribe N, Luu NC, Dmitriev A. Serious complication of low-dose oral minoxidil for hair loss. *JAAD Case Rep.* 2022;30:97–8.

Trüeb RM, Dias MFRG. Alopecia areata: A comprehensive review of pathogenesis and management. *Clin Rev Allergy Immunol.* 2018;54(1):68–87.

Tsai YS, Tong YC, Cheng JT, Lee CH, Yang FS, Lee HY. Pumpkin seed oil and phytosterol-F can block testosterone/prazosin-induced prostate growth in rats. *Urol Int.* 2006;77(3):269–74.

Tyagi V, Singh PK. A new approach to treating scarring alopecia by hair transplantation and topical minoxidil. *Indian J Dermatol Venereol Leprol.* 2010;76(2):215.

U.S. National Library of Medicine, Drug information [internet]; 2024. https://dailymed.nlm.nih.gov/dailymed/drugInfo.cfm?setid=6f904709-65aa-44ce-b144-b4c8a0416e36.

Ubbink DT, Santema TB, Lapid O. Shared decision-making in cosmetic medicine and aesthetic surgery. *Aesthet Surg J.* 2016;36(1):NP14–19.

Udompanich S, Chanprapaph K, Suchonwanit P. Hair and scalp changes in cutaneous and systemic lupus erythematosus. Am J Clin Dermatol. 2018;19(5):679–94.

Uebel CO, da Silva JB, Cantarelli D, Martins P. The role of platelet plasma growth factors in male pattern baldness surgery. *Plast Reconstr Surg.* 2006;118(6):1458–66.

Umar S et al. Treatment-refractory central centrifugal cicatricial alopecia responsive to a novel botanical treatment. *Clin Cosmet Investig Dermatol.* 2022;15:609–19.

van Beek N, Bodó E, Kromminga A, Gáspár E, Meyer K, Zmijewski MA, Slominski A, Wenzel BE, Paus R. Thyroid hormones directly alter human hair follicle functions: Anagen prolongation and stimulation of both hair matrix keratinocyte proliferation and hair pigmentation. *J Clin Endocrinol Metab.* 2008;93(11):4381–88.

Van Delen M, Derdelinckx J, Wouters K, Nelissen I, Cools N. A systematic review and meta-analysis of clinical trials assessing safety and efficacy of human extracellular vesicle-based therapy. *J Extracell Vesicles.* 2024;13(7):e12458.

Van Neste D. Placebo-controlled dose-effect studies with topical minoxidil 2% or 5% in male-patterned hair loss treated with oral finasteride employing an analytical and exhaustive study protocol. *Skin Res Technol.* 2020;26(4):542–57.

Vañó-Galván S, Saceda-Corralo D, Moreno-Arrones OM, Rodrigues-Barata R, Morales C, Gil-Redondo R, Bernárdez-Guerra C, Hermosa-Gelbard Á, Jaén-Olasolo P. Effectiveness and safety of oral dutasteride for male androgenetic alopecia in real clinical practice: A descriptive monocentric study. *Dermatol Ther.* 2020;33(1):e13182.

Vidali S, Knuever J, Lerchner J, Giesen M, Bíró T, Klinger M, Kofler B, Funk W, Poeggeler B, Paus R. Hypothalamic-pituitary-thyroid axis hormones stimulate mitochondrial function and biogenesis in human hair follicles. *J Invest Dermatol.* 2014;134(1):33–42.

Völker JM, Koch N, Becker M, Klenk A. Caffeine and its pharmacological benefits in the management of androgenetic alopecia: A review. *Skin Pharmacol Physiol.* 2020;33(3):93–109.

Wallace ML, Smoller BR. Estrogen and progesterone receptors in androgenic alopecia versus alopecia areata. *Am J Dermatopathol.* 1998;20(2):160–3.

Wambier CG, Craiglow BG, King BA. Combination tofacitinib and oral minoxidil treatment for severe alopecia areata. *J Am Acad Dermatol.* 2019:S0190-9622(19)32688-X.

Wang ECE, Higgins CA. Immune cell regulation of the hair cycle. *Exp Dermatol.* 2020;29(3):322–33.

Wang X, Ramos R, Phan AQ, Yamaga K, Flesher JL, Jiang S, Oh JW, Jin S, Jahid S, Kuan CH, Nguyen TK, Liang HY, Shettigar NU, Hou R, Tran KH, Nguyen A, Vu KN, Phung JL, Ingal JP, Levitt KM, Plikus MV. Signalling by senescent melanocytes hyperactivates hair growth. *Nature.* 2023;618(7966):808–17.

Wang X, Wang H, Xu D, et al. Risk of valproic acid-related alopecia: A systematic review and meta-analysis. *Seizure.* 2019;69:61–9.

Wang Y, Qian H. Phthalates and their impacts on human health. *Healthcare (Basel).* 2021;9(5):603.

Weger N, Schlake T. IGF-I signalling controls the hair growth cycle and the differentiation of hair shafts. *J Invest Dermatol.* 2005;125(5):873–82.

Whiting DA. Chronic telogen effluvium. *Dermatol Clin.* 1996;14(4):723–31.
Williams NM, Randolph M, Rajabi-Estarabadi A, Keri J, Tosti A. Hormonal contraceptives and dermatology. *Am J Clin Dermatol.* 2021;22(1):69–80.
Wirya CT, Wu W, Wu K. Classification of male-pattern hair loss. Int J Trichology. 2017;9(3):95–100.
Wu X, Huang X, Zhu Q, Zhang J, Hu J, Song Y, You Y, Zhu L, Lu J, Xu X, Chen M, Wang W, Song X, Ji J, Du Y. Hybrid hair follicle stem cell extracellular vesicles co-delivering finasteride and gold nanoparticles for androgenetic alopecia treatment. *J Control Release.* 2024;373:652–66.
Xu L, Liu KX, Senna MM. A practical approach to the diagnosis and management of hair loss in children and adolescents. *Front Med (Lausanne).* 2017;4:112.
Yan L, Kageyama T, Zhang B, Yamashita S, Molino PJ, Wallace GG, Fukuda J. Electrical stimulation to human dermal papilla cells for hair regenerative medicine. *J Biosci Bioeng.* 2022;133(3):281–90.
Yan W, Liu J, Xie X, Jin Q, Yang Y, Pan Y, Zhang Y, Zhang F, Wang Y, Liu J, Jin L. Restoration of follicular β-catenin signaling by mesenchymal stem cells promotes hair growth in mice with androgenetic alopecia. *Stem Cell Res Ther.* 2024;15(1):439.
Yang X, Yu W, Qiao R, Sun J, Jiang Y. The predictive value of midscalp hair density and terminal hair percentage in the severity evaluation of FPHL assessed by TrichoScan in a sample of Chinese population. *Clinical, Cosmetic and Investigational Dermatol.* 2022;15:2675—84.
Yepuri V, Venkataram M. Platelet-rich plasma with microneedling in androgenetic alopecia: Study of efficacy of the treatment and the number of sessions required. *J Cutan Aesthet Surg.* 2021;14(2):184–90.
Yimam M, Lee YC, Jiao P, Hong M, Brownell L, Jia Q. A standardized composition comprised of extracts from *Rosmarinus officinalis*, *Annona squamosa*, and *Zanthoxylum clava-herculis* for cellulite. *Pharmacognosy Res.* 2017;9(4):319–24.
Yip L, Rufaut N, Sinclair R. Role of genetics and sex steroid hormones in male androgenetic alopecia and female pattern hair loss: An update of what we now know. *Australas J Dermatol.* 2011;52(2):81–8.
Yip L, Zaloumis S, Irwin D, Severi G, Hopper J, Giles G, et al. Gene-wide association study between the aromatase gene (CYP19A1) and female pattern hair loss. *Br J Dermatol.* 2009;161.
Yuan A, Gu Y, Bian Q, Wang R, Xu Y, Ma X, Zhou Y, Gao J. Conditioned media-integrated microneedles for hair regeneration through perifollicular angiogenesis. *J Control Release.* 2022;350:204–14.
Zakaria W, Passeron T, Ostovari N, Lacour JP, Ortonne JP. 308-nm excimer laser therapy in alopecia areata. *J Am Acad Dermatol.* 2004;51(5):837–8.
Zarei M, Wikramanayake TC, Falto-Aizpurua L, Schachner LA, Jimenez JJ. Low level laser therapy and hair regrowth: an evidence-based review. *Lasers Med Sci.* 2016;31(2):363–71.
Zhang D, LaSenna C, Shields BE. Culprits of medication-induced telogen effluvium, part 1. *Cutis.* 2023 Dec;112(6):267–71.
Zhang H, Yao J, Jiang Q, Shi Y, Ge W, Xu X. Engineered exosomes biopotentiated hydrogel promote hair follicle growth via reprogramming the perifollicular microenvironment. *Pharmaceutics.* 2024;16(7):935.
Zhang S, Zhou H, Chen X, Zhu S, Chen D, Luo D, Chen S, Liu W. Microneedle delivery platform integrated with codelivery nanoliposomes for effective and safe androgenetic alopecia treatment. *ACS Appl Mater Interfaces.* 2024;16(13):15701–17
Zhang W, Guo Y, Kuss M, Shi W, Aldrich AL, Untrauer J, Kielian T, Duan B. Platelet-rich plasma for the treatment of tissue infection: Preparation and clinical evaluation. *Tissue Eng Part B Rev.* 2019;25(3):225–36.
Zhang X, Xiao S, Liu B, Miao Y, Hu Z. Use of extracellular matrix hydrogel from human placenta to restore hair-inductive potential of dermal papilla cells. *Regen Med.* 2019;14(8):741–51.
Zheng W, Xu CH. Innovative approaches and advances for hair follicle regeneration. *ACS Biomater Sci Eng.* 2023;9(5):2251–76. doi:10.1021/acsbiomaterials.3c00028. PMID: 37036820.
Zhou L, Wang H, Jing J, Yu L, Wu X, Lu Z. Regulation of hair follicle development by exosomes derived from dermal papilla cells. *Biochem Biophys Res Commun.* 2018;500(2):325–32.
Zhou Z, Song S, Gao Z, Wu J, Ma J, Cui Y. The efficacy and safety of dutasteride compared with finasteride in treating men with androgenetic alopecia: A systematic review and meta-analysis. *Clin Interv Aging.* 2019;14:399–406.
Zins GR. The history of the development of minoxidil. *Clin Dermatol.* 1988;6(4):132–47.
Żychowska M, Żychowska M. Dermoscopy of discoid lupus erythematosus - a systematic review of the literature. *Int J Dermatol.* 2021;60(7):818–28.

Index

For Product Safety Concerns and Information please contact our EU representative GPSR@taylorandfrancis.com Taylor & Francis Verlag GmbH, Kaufingerstraße 24, 80331 München, Germany

* 9 7 8 1 0 3 2 7 0 5 2 8 6 *

T - #0035 - 181225 - C188 - 254/178/9 [11] - CB - 9781032705286 - Gloss Lamination